CO 1 55

CW00972690

This book is to be returned or

The Family Planning Association
Guide to Contraception

About the Author

SUZIE HAYMAN is an agony aunt, counsellor, author and broadcaster. She is a
member of the National Executive of the
Family Planning Association and is on the
Board of Brook Advisory Centres.

The Family Planning Association Guide to Contraception

SUZIE HAYMAN

Thorsons
An Imprint of HarperCollins*Publishers*

Thorsons
An Imprint of HarperCollins*Publishers*
77–85 Fulham Palace Road,
Hammersmith, London W6 8JB

1160 Battery Street,
San Francisco, California 94111-1213

Published by Thorsons 1993

1 3 5 7 9 10 8 6 4 2

© Suzie Hayman 1993

Suzie Hayman asserts the moral right to
be identified as the author of this work

A catalogue record for this book
is available from the British Library

ISBN 0 7225 2709 8

Typeset by Harper Phototypesetters Limited,
Northampton, England
Printed in Great Britain by
HarperCollinsManufacturing Glasgow

Contents

Introduction: Making Choices

Contraception is all about choices. Whether you call it birth control, fertility control, contraception or family planning, it all adds up to the one idea of *choice*. Contraception can help you choose about making love, making your sexual relationship closer, more exciting and free of worry. Contraception can help you choose about pregnancy, helping you decide if, and exactly when, you are going to start a family and how you will space it. And contraception can help with your sexual health and wider decisions about your well-being and lifestyle. Using contraception puts *you* in control of your body and your life.

If you are going to choose and use a method of contraception, you need information. There are two aspects to finding which methods of contraception may be suitable for you. One is deciding which methods you would feel comfortable and happy using. The other is discovering which methods you might be advised to use, since some methods cannot be used by everyone. This book is designed to help you, by showing you how each method works, how you can use it, how it may affect you and where you can get it, so that you can make your own mind up about what you want to do. But hard facts are not the only consideration when it comes to deciding on the method of birth control that would suit us best. Our feelings are important too – feelings about our sexuality, our sexual relationship, and about whether and when to have children. As well as getting the facts, we need time and opportunity to think and talk them over. So this book will also help you explore what you want from a method of contraception and help you talk over your own opinions and feelings with the people who matter to you or can help you.

The first choice, then, is to find out about the methods available. If you are going to use one, you can then decide which fits in with *your* life, needs, beliefs and tastes. Contraception is like any other consumer product in that you have the right to decide which one you would like to use. As with any other product, what may be right for one person is not necessarily right for another. And as with any other product, there is no one type that is *the* best. Every method has aspects which are particularly useful to some people. The trick is to work out exactly what you want from your method of birth control, because the fact is that a method of contraception works best if you are happy and comfortable with it.

Efficiency may be an important aspect for you. The method used to measure how well a contraceptive method prevents pregnancy is by counting how many women would become pregnant if 100 couples were using it over a period of a year. For instance, between 1 and 3 women out of every 100 become pregnant using an intrauterine device (IUD). So we would say the IUD is 97-99 per cent effective. However, the efficiency of a method may lie as much in the way you use it as in its own in-built action. Some methods *can* be less effective with less committed use, but become extremely efficient if you and your partner use them consistently and according to instructions. For many couples, efficiency may *not* be the strongest consideration. Even if it is important to you not to become pregnant at this particular time, other factors may weigh as heavily in the balance for you.

Whether your method is separate from the act of love can be part of your decision. Some methods should be thought about just before or during lovemaking, some should be remembered daily or once every month or few months. Some methods have a positive, protective effect on certain aspects of your health, or they may increase the chances of your experiencing other health problems. Balancing one against the other may be part of your decision. Some methods are easily and quickly reversible when you want to get pregnant, while using others may mean a slight delay or are intended to make sure you cannot get pregnant again. Some methods require additional use of creams or foams that could increase lubrication, while others hold or soak up sperm, and some need you to touch your own or your partner's genitals. All of these could be seen by some as an enjoyable part of love-making and by others as less acceptable.

Where and how you are going to obtain your contraception may also be a part of your decision making. For some methods you would see a doctor, while others can be bought over the counter. All methods of contraception are free in the UK, if you go to a doctor's surgery or a family planning or youth advisory clinic, but some methods are only available from clinics and there may not be one near you which is open at a convenient time.

All these aspects of a method of contraception are important to us, both as individuals or as part of a couple. Thinking about and then discussing all of these factors with a sexual partner and with a doctor or nurse can help you arrive at a choice that suits you best. There is a wide range of professionals available to you, to help you make a decision and to be on hand to discuss any queries or worries. As well as plenty of methods, there are plenty of people with whom you can discuss your choices. Being able to talk about your needs can help you arrive at the choice that suits you best.

Sometimes you may find it helpful to write your ideas down, when you come to consider which method might suit you. Take a sheet of paper and list all the aspects of birth control that come to mind. Put them in order of importance. If you have a partner, ask him or her to do the same. Then, talk over your views and see if the items and order are different. If so, discuss what differs and why. If you see a doctor or nurse about contraception, take the list with you and use it to talk over your needs and feelings about contraception.

There are currently many basic methods of contraception, with quite a few variations within several of the methods. This

gives you plenty of choice and plenty of chances to find
something that suits you and your partner. It is also important
to note that your needs may change at different points in your
life. It might at times be particularly important that you be fully
protected against pregnancy, but at other stages you may not
mind so much if a pregnancy came along. You may sometimes
need protection against sexual infections, but at others, when
you and your partner are in a mutually faithful relationship,
such concerns may not be necessary. As you get older your
fertility decreases so that you feel happy about using methods
that may not have seemed efficient enough at an earlier stage,
and methods that might not have seemed convenient or
suitable become more acceptable. So, having chosen a
method, it is worth keeping your options open and recog-
nizing that you may wish to use something else at another
time.

You may be reading this book in preparation for trying
contraception for the first time, or you may already be an
established user but interested in a different method from the
one you use now. Whatever your situation, it is hoped that you
find something of use in the following chapters. Of course, this
book can only summarize the information about methods of
contraception based on evidence available and current medical
opinion at the time of publication. This book does not replace
information from your doctor or the manufacturer's packet
information.

CHAPTER ONE

Pregnancy

We have looked at the concept of choice – when, why and how do we make decisions about our fertility? The next stage is to look at the various methods we can choose between, if our decision *is* to use a form of birth control, now or in the future, and our options if an unplanned pregnancy is begun. For you to make a fully-informed choice, you need to understand how contraception works, and that is what the rest of this book is all about. But to do that, it may help to first consider how *conception* happens.

We call the parts of the body that are involved in having sex and making a pregnancy the reproductive organs. The outer sexual parts of the body are called the genitals.

The Female Reproductive Organs

In the woman, this area is known as the vulva. Soft folds of skin surround two openings – the urethra, through which you pass urine, and the vagina. These fleshy folds are called labia – the Latin for 'lips'. The inner pair or labia minora – small lips – are hairless and fairly shiny. The outer sides of the labia majora – large lips – are usually covered in hair. Labia often appear somewhat coarse in texture and frilly or wrinkled at the edges. Both sets can be small and neat or long, hanging down quite a way. Just as hands, feet or faces vary in size and shape from person to person, so labia vary in size and appearance in different people.

To the front of the vulva, the labia minora join and form a hood, protecting the clitoris. This small nub of flesh is the most sensitive, sexy area in a woman and the main site of sexual pleasure. Behind the clitoris is the opening to the urethra, usually hidden by the labia, which touch each other when a woman has her legs together. Behind the opening to the urethra, also concealed unless the labia are parted, is the opening of the vagina.

The vagina is a flexible tube which slants into the body, along a line drawn from the vulva towards the small of the back. The vagina is at its narrowest in the first few centimetres of its

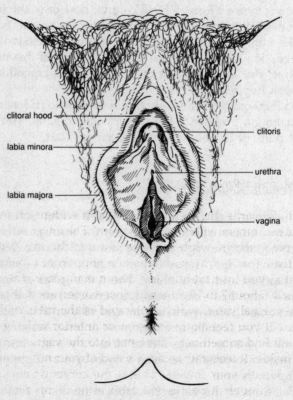

clitoral hood

clitoris

labia minora

urethra

labia majora

vagina

Figure 1: External female sex organs

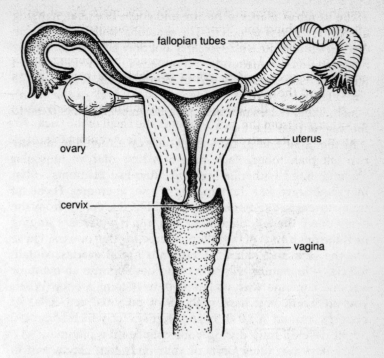

Figure 2: Internal female sex organs

length. Towards the upper two thirds, it widens and during sexual excitement will even 'balloon out'. The lower third is rich in nerve endings, while the area towards the top is far less sensitive. That is why you can feel a tampon or a diaphragm or cap as you insert it but not when it is in place. The vagina is usually about 7 to 10 cm long. Most women are able to reach to the vaginal vault, which is the end of the tube, with their fingers. If you feel along the front or anterior wall, however, you will find something jutting out into the vagina some 6 to 8 cm inside. It feels rather like the end of your nose when you touch it with your fingers. This is the cervix or neck of the womb. Through it passes the cervical os or opening to the womb.

The womb or uterus is the size and shape of a pear, hanging upside down in your pelvis. The muscular walls of the womb can stretch to quite a size to carry not only a developing baby but the fluid that surrounds and protects it. The womb is lined with soft tissue, which is rich in blood vessels. It is about 7.5 cm long, but a third of this length is the neck of the womb which, like the stem of that upside-down pear, points out into the vagina near the top.

At the other end of the womb, one on either side, are the two fallopian tubes. Each tube is a tiny, narrow, muscular channel, lined with cilia – minute hair-like filaments – that move and wave, like the tentacles of a sea anemone. These set up a current in fluids moving around in the pelvis, from the ovary down the fallopian tubes and into the uterus. Hanging near the open ends of the fallopian tubes are the ovaries. These are the size and shape of almonds. Your ovaries contain follicles – immature cells that could develop into an ovum or egg and combine with male sperm to become a baby. When you are born, you have millions of potential egg cells. At puberty, around 200,000 follicles remain, of which some 400 might develop fully during your childbearing lifetime.

You have two other parts of your body that play a part in controlling your menstrual cycle and your chances of getting pregnant. One is the hypothalamus, which is a part of the brain. The other is the pituitary, which is a gland at the base of the brain. The hypothalamus sends out chemicals which act as messengers. They tell the pituitary to make hormones, which are also chemical messengers. It is these that drive your menstrual cycle. Each month, you release an egg (ovulation) and will have a period because of the rise and fall of hormones. The changes that take place in your body that lead to a monthly bleed can also lead to a pregnancy.

The Menstrual Cycle

Each month, the pituitary will start the menstrual cycle by producing a hormone called follicle-stimulating hormone (FSH). This triggers ten or twenty follicles to begin to ripen in your ovaries. As these grow, the follicles themselves produce a second hormone, oestrogen. This acts on the lining of the womb, causing it to thicken and grow in preparation for a fertilized egg. After 6 to 8 days, the pituitary stops producing FSH and makes luteinizing hormone (LH) instead. This stimulates one of the follicles to burst open on the surface of the ovary and to release an ovum or egg. This is ovulation, a woman's most fertile time, which occurs 12 to 16 days *before* your next period. Each ovary usually takes it in turn to release an egg. Usually, only one follicle will mature, but sometimes two sites burst open at the same time. If both these eggs are fertilized and come to a full-term pregnancy, the result would be non-identical twins.

The egg, when released, will be caught in the current of fluid pulled from the cavity and down the fallopian tubes by the tiny, waving hair-like cells. The egg is at its best in the first 12 hours after ovulation, although it can survive for up to 24 hours. If it is to be fertilized, it needs to meet living, vigorous sperm almost as soon as it enters the fallopian tube. If sperm is not encountered at the right time in the journey from ovary to womb, the egg will not be fertilized and will be washed out of the body in the normal flow of fluid. If sperm is waiting in the tube or arrives soon after, it will surround the egg and one sperm will break through the egg's covering. This is fertilization. The male cell and the female cell will combine and the resultant bundle of cells, called a blastocyst, will continue down to the womb. The egg would take around seven to eight days to complete that journey.

After the egg has burst out of the ovary, the follicle it has left becomes the 'corpus luteum', or yellow body, named for its colour. This makes yet another hormone as well as oestrogen – progesterone. Progesterone prevents any more eggs being released, which is why you can't get pregnant again while you are already carrying a baby. The fertilized egg will arrive in the womb and will embed in the thick, rich and welcoming lining, where it will continue to grow and develop. This is called implantation. Once implanted, an egg passes a hormone called human chorionic gonadotrophin (HCG) into the woman's bloodstream. This keeps up the body's production of progesterone, which sends signals to your body to maintain the lining of the womb and to keep the pregnancy going. If the lining or endometrium is not ready or hormone levels are at the wrong stage, the egg will not implant.

If the egg is not fertilized, the corpus luteum shrinks and stops producing progesterone, some 12 to 16 days after ovulation. The lining of the womb starts to disintegrate in response to the lack of progesterone. It then comes away as a flow of blood, tissue and fluid – your period. The amount you lose can be from 50 to 175 cc – around a quarter to three-quarters of a cup. The womb does not 'store up' blood. If your period is a little heavier than usual one month, it will be because the lining has grown thicker for that month, not because blood has been blocked or held back inside you. A light period is a result of the lining having been thinner in that month. As you bleed, FSH levels will begin to pick up, starting the whole cycle over again.

For convenience we tend to talk about the menstrual cycle as a month or 28 days. In fact, the normal range – from first day of bleeding to the last day before the next bleed – can be from 21 to 35 days, with an average spread of 25 to 30 days.

The Male Reproductive Organs

In the man, the genitals consist of the penis, which is made up of soft, spongy tissue and veins, and the testicles, which hang below and behind the penis inside the scrotum, which is a soft bag of skin and tissue. The testicles are similar to the woman's ovaries: they are glands which make sperm. Unlike

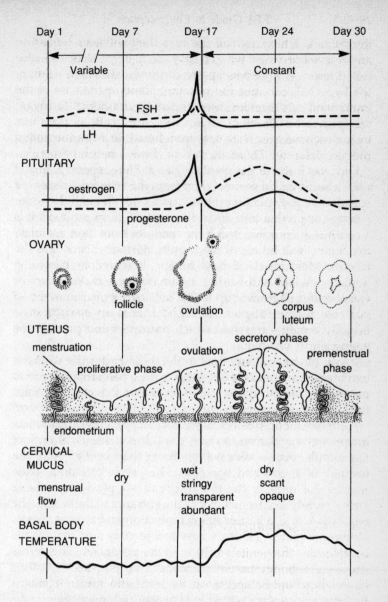

Figure 3: The menstrual cycle

the ovaries, which have all the eggs they will ever contain in an undeveloped state when a baby girl is born, testicles – also called testes – make new sperm continuously. As in women, the hypothalamus and the pituitary gland at the base of the brain send out chemical messengers or hormones to trigger this process. Millions of sperm cells are made all the time, inside each testicle. They pass from here into a channel called the vas deferens. There are two of these, one on each side.

Each vas leads to the prostate gland. Here, sperm is mixed with a liquid called seminal fluid from the seminal vesicles. At ejaculation, the resulting semen passes out through the water passage or urethra and down the penis. Sperm production is a continuous process, and if the man does not have a climax, his semen will be reabsorbed, quite normally, back into the tissues. Most men will pass semen, however, by becoming sexually excited and having a climax. Each male climax or ejaculation will contain up to 300 million sperm. However, 98 per cent of the teaspoon of liquid that is an ejaculation is actually semen – the fluid which nourishes and protects the sperm on its journey.

If you have sex at any time in the month near the woman's ovulation, you could set in motion the process that leads to pregnancy. Since sperm travel at about 2.5 cm per hour, fertilization can happen some 10 to 12 hours after sex. Sperm can survive for up to seven days, but can probably only fertilize a woman's egg for up to three days. If it is the right time of the month, your bodies will be doing their best to make the journey of sperm and egg easy. The cervix produces fertile mucus. For most of the month the cervix produces a thick, sticky, cloudy mucus that blocks the entrance to the womb (the os). This acts as a barrier against infection and against sperm. Around ovulation (12 to 16 days before your next period) the cervix will soften and produce far more mucus. This fertile mucus is clear and stretchy. Instead of plugging the os, it forms channels to speed sperm on its way. The mucus contains proteins and sugars which feed sperm on its journey.

Your body is programmed to try for a pregnancy, but does

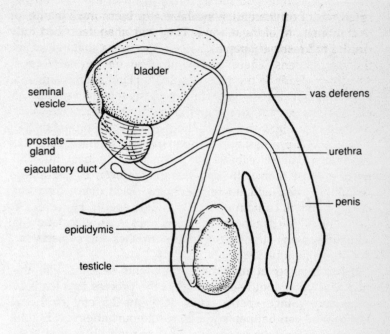

Figure 4: Male sex organs

not always succeed. Not every egg that is released is fertilized, and a high proportion of fertilized eggs quite naturally and normally fail to implant or are rejected by the body after implantation. This is why it can take a couple who are in good health, of average fertility and having regular sex, up to 18 months before succeeding with a pregnancy.

However, there is always the possibility that any act of unprotected sex *could* result in conception. Having looked at how a pregnancy can be started, you can see how conception may be stopped by:

1 preventing ovulation
2 preventing the meeting of egg and sperm
3 immobilizing or killing sperm.

Methods of contraception available at present work in one, or a combination, of these ways. They will all be described fully in the following chapters.

CHAPTER TWO

Hormonal Contraception

Your body makes its own hormones, two of which, oestrogen and progesterone, drive your menstrual cycle and are involved both in beginning and in maintaining a pregnancy. Hormonal contraception prevents pregnancy by using synthetic versions of these natural hormones. These work by stopping ovulation, thickening cervical mucus to make a barrier to sperm, causing the lining of the womb to be thin and inhospitable to a fertilized egg, or a combination of these factors. Hormonal contraception is delivered in a measured dose of hormones to your body. This can be done by having you take a pill by mouth, as a daily dose. Or you can use an implant, an injection or a vaginal ring, when the hormones are gradually and continuously absorbed.

Ovulation is prevented when these hormones give chemical messages to your hypothalamus and your pituitary gland, which produce the hormones that tell your ovaries what to do. Instead of being triggered into maturing, follicles in the ovaries do not ripen and no eggs are released to be fertilized.

Hormonal contraception also encourages cervical mucus to be thick and sticky. This acts as a barrier, plugging the entrance to the womb and stopping sperm from swimming up into the fallopian tubes. This mucus is quite acidic and this may also make the sperm sluggish and slow. Hormonal contraception affects the fallopian tubes, too. Instead of wafting a matured egg on its way to meet a sperm, the fallopian tubes slow this journey down. If an egg *does* meet up with a sperm and *is* fertilized, it then takes too long to reach the womb to be at the right stage to be welcomed. The lining of the womb itself will also be too thin and poor for a fertilized egg to implant and develop.

Oral Contraception

Also known as the Pill.

'The contraceptive you can eat' was the headline that greeted oral contraception when it first became available. This seemed a novel idea at a time. It was hardly new, however. Women through the ages have taken herbal potions intended to stop a pregnancy or cause a miscarriage. But scientists needed to understand the part the hormones oestrogen and progesterone played in the menstrual cycle, conception and pregnancy, before modern oral contraception could be developed. After trials in 1956, the first Pill was made available in the United States in 1959. It was first used in Britain in 1961.

There are two basic types of oral contraception – the combined pill which contains oestrogen and progestogen (synthetic progesterone), and the progestogen-only pill.

The Combined Pill

The combined pill works mainly by preventing ovulation. It also encourages cervical mucus to form a barrier to sperm. In addition, it alters the movement of the fallopian tubes to slow the journey of sperm and egg and makes the lining of the womb thinner and therefore inhospitable.

At present, the Pill is the most popular method of contraception in the UK. Around three million women (23 per cent of those aged between 16 and 49) use it. Worldwide, about 50 million women rely on the Pill for birth control. Half of these are living in developed countries such as the United States, or in the European Community where between 15 and 30 per cent of women able to get pregnant are using the Pill. In developing countries, five or six per cent of women of childbearing age are Pill users.

The combined pill is a very effective method of contraception. Taken without any mistakes or mishaps, your chances of becoming pregnant while using it are practically nil. However, between 0.1 and seven out of every 100 women taking the combined pill for a year *do* get pregnant. Most combined pill failures are caused by users missing pills, or having something happen to them or doing something they had not realized would prevent their pills working. The more you understand about how the Pill works and the more you feel in control, the less likely you are to be let down by it.

How Do You Use The Combined Pill?

Combined pills come in 'bubble' or 'blister' packs – flat oblongs or circular packs with the pills visible through one side. You press the pills out through the other side which is made of thin foil. The packets are printed so that each pill is marked with the day of the week, with an arrow leading you round from Monday through the week to Sunday and so on. Most combined pills come in packets of 21, although some (ED or Everyday combined pills) are in packets of 28.

There are three types of combined pills – monophasic, biphasic and triphasic. Monophasic means 'one-step'. In these, each pill in the packet contains exactly the same balance of oestrogen and progestogen. Biphasic means 'two-step', and in these the first seven pills have less progestogen than the remaining 14. Triphasic means 'three-step' and there are three different phases of pills in each packet. In packets of biphasic

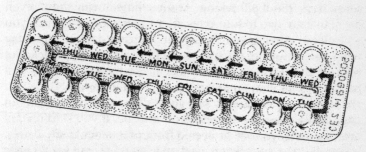

Figure 5: The Combined Pill – one of many brands available

and triphasic pills, the sets of pills have a different colour so that you can tell them apart and take them in the correct order. This is because if you made a mistake and took a pill out of sequence it would not matter if you were taking a monophasic pill, or a pill from the same phase of bi- or triphasic pills, but it might matter if you got the wrong set and therefore the wrong formula of bi- or triphasic pills.

Using The Combined Pill

To take the combined pill, you begin by taking your first pill on the first day – or day one – of a period. In fact, you can start the pill on any day during your cycle. However, starting during a period ensures there is no possibility that you could be already pregnant at the time. It is now normal, in the UK, to start the pill on the first day of bleeding. If you were taking the combined pill, that day becomes your 'starting day.' Let's say it is a Thursday. You will then take a pill each day for three weeks. It doesn't matter what time of the day you chose to do this, but it is important to pick a time you can remember and stick to. You mustn't be more than 12 hours late taking any pill, or contraceptive protection is lost. That means you can't let more than 36 hours go between pills. Having taken the last pill in the packet (it will be on the day of the week before your 'starting day' – a Wednesday in this case) you will then have seven days free of pill-taking. At some time during those seven days, usually two to four days after finishing that packet, you will bleed. After seven days your 'starting day' of Thursday will come round again and you will begin another packet of pills. It is important to note that it is only on the very *first* packet of pills that you start on day 1 of a period. Once you are taking the combined pill you follow a 21 days on/seven days off/21 days on/seven days off routine. If you start on day one of a cycle, you are protected from pregnancy immediately. If you did start your first packet on a later day, you would have to use another method of contraception, such as the condom, for the first seven days (14 days for ED pills) of taking your first packet. When taking the pill, you are protected from pregnancy for your entire cycle – including the seven 'pill free' days, as long as you begin the next packet on time.

Some people find having seven days off makes them forget to start their next packet on time. To help avoid this, there are combined pills that come in packets of 28. Seven of the pills are 'placebos' or inactive sugar pills. They are there simply to help you stay in the habit of taking a pill every day. With this type, called Everyday combined pills or ED pills, having taken your very first pill of your first packet on day 1 of a period, you take a pill every day and go straight from the end of one packet to the beginning of another. But it *is* important to follow the arrows round and not get out of sequence.

Missing Pills

If you miss a pill or take one too late, you will be at risk of pregnancy.

The worst combined pills to miss are those at the beginning or the end of each packet. In ED pills, the worst ones to miss are those at either side of the 'inactive' pills. If you missed out one of those, you lengthen the time you go without a combined pill to over seven days and this may allow an egg to be released. If you do forget a pill, take it as soon as you realize what has happened, and take the rest of your pills as usual. If you are less than 12 hours late, you will still be protected from pregnancy. If you are more than 12 hours late you should abstain from sex or use another method of contraception (such as the condom) *as well* for the next seven days. If you find that this seven days takes you into your pill-free week, leave out the break. Go straight on to starting a new packet and take them as usual. You will get a bleed at the end of this second packet. If you are taking the ED pill, and are more than 12 hours late in taking it, you should use another method for the next seven days. If this takes you into the seven 'inactive' pills, miss them out, throw the packet away and go straight on to another packet of pills. Missing a break in this way is not at all harmful to you. Your next period will come at the end of the second packet, or while you are taking the inactive pills with ED pills. Some women may get some breakthrough bleeding after missing a pill at some point during the second packet. If you do get breakthrough bleeding you shouldn't worry as it isn't harmful, and doesn't mean there is a problem.

You need to take the combined pill exactly as recommended for it to work. If you miss a pill or two or are late starting a new packet, it simply won't work. If this does happen, and you have not followed the instructions for 'missing pills', see your doctor at once to discuss your options, such as emergency contraception. If you are having doubts or any worries about using oral contraception, don't stop taking your pills in mid-packet. See your doctor first to talk over any concerns and to discuss other options.

However, even if you are taking the combined pill according to the instructions, there are other things that can happen to you that may affect its ability to protect you from pregnancy.

The combined pill needs to be in your body long enough for it to be taken into your system properly. If you vomit before a pill has been absorbed, you have, in effect, missed a pill. If you are sick within three hours of taking a pill, you need to take another pill straight away. If you go on being sick, you need to wait until you are well enough to keep your pill down and then go back to your usual routine. You would be at risk of pregnancy all the time you were being sick and up until seven days after you went back to regular pill-taking again. So you would have to use another method of birth control during this time and follow the advice given above for 'missing pills'.

You have the same problem if you suffer *very severe* diarrhoea within 12 hours of taking your pill. You should keep taking the pill as normal, but you should use another method of birth control while you are unwell, and for seven days after the last day of illness. Follow the advice given above for 'missing pills.'

It is also worth noting that anything that 'hurries along' your food may have the same effect. Taking purgatives or laxatives while on the pill may alter the way the pill is absorbed. It would depend on how often you took them, the amount you used and at what stage in your pill-taking. If you do take either of these, it would be a good idea to talk it over with your doctor.

Certain drugs you might be given by a doctor at a surgery or hospital, or by a dentist, could also stop the combined pill working properly. Some antibiotics, some prescribed pain-killers, tranquillizers, anti-convulsants and anti-fungal treat-ments (tablets taken for skin and nail infections) are among the treatments that have this effect, if you are using the combined pill.

Some drugs are themselves affected by the combined pill. Your doctor should have the full list of treatments that affect or are affected by it. Even if you have been given the combined pill by your own GP, always remind them of the fact that you are using it when you are given a prescription. And if you are getting your pills through another doctor, tell your own GP if he or she doesn't already know this. You can also check with the pharmacist when you get a prescription. Your doctor can then discuss with you how long you might be unprotected while taking a course of treatment and could help you with other precautions for this period.

Can I Use The Combined Pill?

Healthy women can take the combined pill all their child-bearing lives. However, if you smoke or are overweight, you may be advised to stop and consider another method of contraception around the age of 35. It is no longer suggested that women should have a break every two years or so from pill-taking. There is no medical reason for this and in the past it actually often resulted in unwanted pregnancy. In fact, if you are using a combined pill, you already have 13 natural breaks every year each time you pause between one packet and the next or take the sugar pills in your Everyday packet.

Before prescribing a combined pill, the nurse or doctor will ask you about your health and that of your immediate family. This is because the combined pill may make some conditions worse. These conditions include certain illnesses affecting your cardiovascular system – that is, your heart and blood supply – or your liver; some gynaecological conditions; cancers affecting the reproductive organs; some metabolic or hormonal problems. The doctor will also need to know if you smoke, have severe depression or severe migraine. The doctor may advise you not to take a combined pill but to consider an alternative method.

Your weight and blood pressure will be measured and you will be offered a vaginal examination and a smear test. If, after completing the necessary physical checks and discussion, your doctor agrees that combined oral contraception would be suitable for you, you will be given a prescription or supplies. You will be asked to return for a follow-up check, usually in three months. If there were no problems at that stage, you will then be given supplies for a longer period and asked to return at regular intervals for routine health checks. If you have any problems or worries, you can of course return at any time.

Advantages of the Combined Pill

The combined pill is convenient and easy to use and does not interfere with lovemaking. Many couples find that their sex life improves when they use it as their method of contraception. They may be able to show their love more often and spontaneously than before, with fear of pregnancy removed.

The combined pill can help with periods, making them shorter, lighter, less painful and more regular. Used properly, the combined pill is one of the most effective methods of birth control. You can take the combined pill secure in the knowledge that when you stop, you have the same chance of having a healthy pregnancy and baby than if you had never taken it. It can be used by a woman who has never had a pregnancy or it can be started on day 21 after a baby is born, if you are not breastfeeding, and immediately after a miscarriage or an abortion. Being on the combined pill protects you against quite a few conditions, including:

cancer of the endometrium (lining of the womb)

cancer of the ovaries

ovarian cysts

pelvic inflammatory disease (PID)

fibroids

endometriosis

anaemia

polycystic ovary syndrome

heavy, painful periods and premenstrual syndrome

some benign (non-cancerous) breast tumours.

There are a very large number of oral contraceptive pills, made up of different combinations of oestrogen and progestogen, available at the moment. This provides quite a choice, depending on your emotional and medical needs. For instance, if you have a tendency to have acne, some pills would be better than others. There is even a pill – Dianette – that is only prescribed by GPs for treating acne but that is also a contraceptive. When you see your doctor to discuss oral contraception, do remember to tell him or her if you are concerned about such problems.

Disadvantages of the Combined Pill

To be an effective contraceptive, the combined pill has to be taken regularly. You always need to see a doctor or trained medical professional to get it, and some women can't take oral contraceptives for health reasons. There are risks of side effects and some medical problems.

Side Effects of the Combined Pill

There can be no doubt that many women experience side effects when taking the combined pill. *All* drugs have side effects, some bad and some good. However, many of us may experience side effects on the combined pill because we *expect* to do so. In one study, women were given dummy pills, without being aware they were not real pills, before going on real ones. Side effects were reported most often in the month *before* a single real pill had been taken. This doesn't mean that side effects are all in the mind. Side effects can be as genuine as they are unpleasant. But your own concerns or unease could encourage them to happen and make you less able to put up with any discomfort. You may also blame something on the combined pill that actually has another cause. Being on the combined pill often becomes a convenient 'explanation' for all sorts of unpleasant experiences. When side effects do occur, they usually only last for the first month or two and then pass, but **do** discuss any concerns you have with your doctor or clinic instead of just stopping taking the pills – a different pill may not have the unwanted effects.

It is not unusual to feel nauseous at any time during the first three packets, but especially at the beginning of each packet, or first thing when you wake up. Some women find it helps to take the combined pill with the last meal of your day. Some studies show that reduced sexual feelings and depression may occur in some women on the combined pill. Headaches are often mentioned as a side effect when taking the combined pill, either during the three weeks on it or in the seven-day pill-free period.

Some women do say their hair becomes thinner while taking it, while others say the Pill improves hair quality, just as in pregnancy. Thrush can be a problem, although this tended to be an effect with the older pills, not with today's low-dose combined pills.

Some women put on weight in the early months of starting the combined pill. This is partly due to the hormones making you feel hungry, which may result in changes in your eating or exercising behaviour. The same hormones also encourage fluid retention. Today's combined pills are less likely to produce weight gain, but women who do have a tendency to put on weight should make an effort to watch their diet and to do some additional exercise to help keep a balance. Any increase in weight is usually lost after the third packet but if it is not, return to your doctor or clinic and discuss the situation.

Some women experience *chloasma* or brown patches appearing on the skin during pregnancy. This may also happen to such women if they go on the Pill. These patches are particularly noticeable on the face and neck. They may darken slowly over a period of time, but speed up if you are in bright sunlight. Since chloasma often runs in families, you may be able to tell if you might be prone by finding out if a blood-related female relative – your mother, grandmother, aunt or sister – experienced it while on the combined pill or during pregnancy. The patches may fade if you stop taking the combined pill, as they would after a pregnancy, but some trace could remain.

You should note any unpleasant side effects and report them to your doctor. You may need to wait to see if these effects pass, or to try a different pill.

Risks of the Combined Pill
The combined pill may increase your risks of experiencing:

> heart attack (myocardial infarction)
>
> stroke
>
> high blood pressure (hypertension)
>
> blood clot in a vein (thromboembolism)
>
> some liver disease – extremely rare.

However, it is important to get these risks into perspective. In the case of heart attack and stroke, for instance, it is smoking and the combined pill that increases the risk rather than the combined pill on its own. A family history of these problems, occurring before the age of 45, is also important. If you are under 35 and/or a non-smoker and have no other reason to be at risk, being on the combined pill may actually be *safer* than not being on it. The health risks from the combined pill are less than those of an unplanned pregnancy, and overall the combined pill has more of a protective effect than a potentially harmful one. It is important to recognize that today's pills are very much lower in the doses of oestrogen and progestogen than were the early pills. Many of the 'pill scare' stories you may have heard relate to these higher dose pills.

Pregnancy and Breastfeeding and the Combined Pill

The combined pill does not affect your ability to get pregnant after you stop taking it or to have a healthy baby, although some women experience a short delay in getting pregnant immediately after coming off it. Studies show that fewer women get pregnant in the first three months after coming off the combined pill than women who have not been taking it, but this difference evens out after two years. However, women can become pregnant just by missing one pill, or you could stop taking it and get pregnant immediately.

If you do want to plan a pregnancy, it is a good idea to come off the combined pill a month before wanting to start a baby, and to use another method of contraception, such as the condom, until you have a period. This allows the body to return to its pre-pill state and for the pregnancy to be dated more accurately.

Your developing baby will not be affected because you have been on the combined pill. Studies show that women who have become pregnant while taking it or immediately after coming off it are no more likely to suffer miscarriage, ectopic pregnancy or stillbirth or to have a baby with disabilities than women who have never used the Pill.

Neither do you have anything to worry about if a mother-to-be takes the combined pill during the first few weeks, or even longer, of a pregnancy because she doesn't realize she is pregnant. She should stop as soon as she knows she is pregnant, but many studies have shown no increase in abnormalities or problems to babies born when this happens.

Anything a mother eats or drinks while breastfeeding may be passed to her baby through her breast milk. Studies show that babies whose mothers are using the combined pill do take in a very small amount of its hormones during breastfeeding. This has *not* been shown to cause illness or to have any effect on the child's normal development and growth. But since the combined pill also reduces milk flow, women are advised to use another method of contraception while breastfeeding.

The Progestogen-Only Pill

The progestogen-only pill mainly works by acting on cervical mucus, making it thick and encouraging it to form a barrier to sperm. In addition, it alters the movement of the fallopian tubes to slow the journey of sperm and egg and makes the lining of the womb thinner, to prevent fertilization and implantation. Ovulation is prevented in four out of 10 menstrual cycles.

Although the Pill is the most popular method of contraception in the UK, the progestogen-only pill is not as popular as the combined pill. Less than 10 per cent of Pill users – around 300,000 women – take this type. This may be because it is less well-known and is often not offered to women.

Taken without any mistakes or mishaps, less than one in 100 women using this method for a year will become pregnant. With less careful use, between one and four women out of 100 may become pregnant. However, the guidelines for taking the progestogen-only pill correctly are fairly strict, so mistakes can be made that put you at risk of pregnancy. The more you understand about how the progestogen-only pill works and the more you feel in control, the less likely you are to be let down by it. It is worth noting that recent studies indicate that

the failure rate of the progestogen-only pill is higher in women
weighing over 70 kilograms (11 stones).

How Do You Use the Progestogen-Only Pill?

Progestogen-only pills come in 'bubble' or 'blister' packs –
usually flat oblongs with the pills visible through one side. You
press the pills out through the other side, which is made of
thin foil. The packets are printed so that each pill is marked
with the day of the week, and an arrow leading you round
from Monday through the week to Sunday and so on.
Progestogen-only pills come in packets of 28 or 35.

Using The Progestogen-Only Pill

You begin using the Pill by taking your first pill on the first day
– or day one – of a period. You *could* start this at any time in
the cycle, but it is advisable to start on day one of a period,
to make sure you are not pregnant at the time. Once you have
started taking these pills, you simply go on taking one every
day, without a break. Because the progestogen-only pill relies
on changes in cervical mucus and these changes taper off after
the end of the 24-hour period after taking your pill, the birth
control effect quickly wears off. So it is very important to take
a progestogen-only pill at the same time each day, or at least
within three hours of that time. You should not let more than
27 hours go between taking pills, or protection is lost.

If you want the progestogen-only pill to have the best
opportunity of working for you, it is important to find a time
that suits you to take the pill and that enables you to remember
to take it each day. If need be, buy a watch with an alarm, set
it, and take your pill when it rings. If you begin your pill on
day one of a cycle, you are protected immediately.

Missing Pills

If you miss a pill, or are more than three hours late taking one, you could be at risk of pregnancy. You should take your pill as soon as you discover you are late and take the next one at the correct time, and then continue taking your pills at your regular time each day. You should use another method of contraception as well, for the next seven days.

You need to take the progestogen-only pill exactly as recommended for it to work. If you miss a pill or two or are late starting a new packet, it simply won't work. If this does happen, and you have not followed the instructions for 'missing pills,' see your doctor at once to discuss your options, such as emergency contraception. If you are having doubts or any worries about using oral contraception, don't stop taking your pills in mid-packet. See your doctor first to talk over any concerns and to discuss other options.

However, even if you are taking the progestogen-only pill according to the instructions, there are other things that can happen to you that may affect its ability to protect you from pregnancy. The progestogen-only pill needs to be in your body long enough for it to be taken into your system properly. If you vomit before a pill has been absorbed, you have in effect missed a pill. If you are sick within three hours of taking a pill, you need to take another pill straight away. If you go on being sick, you need to wait until you are well enough to keep your pill down and then go back to your usual routine. You are at risk of pregnancy all the time you are being sick and up until seven days after you go back to regular pill-taking again. So you will have to use another method of contraception during this time and follow the advice given above for 'missing pills'.

You have the same problem if you suffer *very severe* diarrhoea within 12 hours of taking your pill. You should keep taking the pill as normal, but you should use another method of birth control while you are unwell, and for seven days after the last day of illness and follow the advice given above for 'missing pills'. It is also worth noting that anything that 'hurries along' your food may have the same effect. Taking purgatives or laxatives while on the progestogen-only pill may alter the way the pill is absorbed. It would depend on how often you took them and the amount you used. If you do take either of these, it would be a good idea to talk it over with your doctor.

Certain drugs you might be given by a doctor at a surgery or hospital, or by a dentist, could also stop the progestogen-only pill working properly. Barbiturates, some prescribed anti-inflammatory drugs, some anti-depressants and drugs that prevent blood clots can affect the progestogen-only pill in this way. Antibiotics do not affect progestogen-only pills.

Some drugs are themselves affected by the progestogen-only pill. Your doctor should have the full list of treatments that affect or are affected by it. Even if you have been given the Pill by your own GP, always remind him or her of the fact that you are using it when you are given a prescription for any other drug. And if you are getting your pills through another doctor, tell your own GP if he or she doesn't already know this. You can also check with the pharmacist when you get a prescription. Your doctor can then discuss with you how long you might be unprotected while taking a course of treatment and could help you with other precautions for this period.

Can I Use the Progestogen-Only Pill?

Progestogen-only pills can be used for the whole of your fertile life, even by some women who are advised not to take the combined pill.

It is no longer suggested that women should have a break every two years or so from pill-taking. There is no medical reason for this and in the past it actually often resulted in unwanted pregnancy.

Before prescribing a contraceptive pill, the nurse or doctor will ask you about your health and that of your immediate family. This is because the Pill may make some conditions worse. Some medical conditions such as cancer of the breast or vagina, active liver disease or severe arterial disease would rule you out. So would having had an ectopic pregnancy – where an egg lodges in and starts to grow in a fallopian tube instead of in the womb. But many of the women who can't take the combined pill *can* take the progestogen-only kind. Doctors often forget about this alternative choice, so if you ask to be 'put on the Pill' and your doctor tells you it would be ill-advised, it is always worth asking *specifically* about the progestogen-only type. If, however, you may find it difficult to take the pill at the same time every day, this method may not be for you.

If, after completing the necessary physical checks and discussion, your doctor agrees that the progestogen-only pill is suitable for you, you will be given a prescription or supplies. You will be asked to return for a follow-up check, usually in three months. If there were no problems at that stage, you will then be given supplies for a longer period and asked to return at regular intervals for routine health checks. If you have any problems or worries, you can of course return at any time.

Advantages of the Progestogen-Only Pill

The progestogen-only pill is convenient and easy to use and does not interfere with lovemaking. Many couples find that their sex life improves when they use it as their method of contraception. They may be able to show their love more often and spontaneously than before, with fear of pregnancy removed.

You can become pregnant quickly and easily after having come off the progestogen-only pill. It is very effective, doesn't stop you breastfeeding and you can start taking it on day 21 after a baby has been born. It can also be started immediately after you have had an abortion or a miscarriage. There are few side effects. Unlike the combined pill, the progestogen-only pill has no link with heart or circulation disease. It can be taken by women who are over 35 and smoke or might be at risk of circulatory diseases. Medical problems, such as high blood pressure and severe diabetes, which would bar you from using a combined pill may not stop you using the progestogen-only pill. Painful periods and PMS may be improved by the progestogen-only pill.

Disadvantages of the Progestogen-Only Pill

To be an effective contraceptive, the progestogen-only pill has to be taken regularly. The progestogen-only pill, particularly, must be taken to a strict timetable, since leaving more than 27 hours between pills may lead to a pregnancy. You always need to see a doctor or trained medical professional to get the pill, and some women can't take oral contraceptives for health reasons.

There are risks of side effects and some medical problems. The progestogen-only pill can upset your periods and is slightly less effective than the combined pill.

Side Effects of the Progestogen-Only Pill
There can be no doubt that many women experience side effects when taking the progestogen-only pill. *All* drugs have side effects, some bad and some good. However, many of us may experience side effects on the progestogen-only pill because we *expect* to do so. This doesn't mean that side effects are all in the mind. Side effects can be as genuine as they are unpleasant. But your own concerns or unease could encourage them to happen and make you less able to put up with any discomfort. You may also blame something on the Pill that actually has another cause. Being on the Pill often becomes a convenient 'explanation' for all sorts of unpleasant experiences. When side effects do occur, they usually only last for the first month or two and then pass, but do discuss any concerns you have with your doctor or clinic, and don't just stop taking the pills.

Some women have headaches, gain weight or lose sexual

urges using the progestogen-only pill. This usually only happens in the first three or four months. Tenderness in the breasts, leg cramps, dizziness and depression are possible, too. Period disturbances, however, are very common, and periods are likely to become irregular. You may also have 'spotting' – when a few drops of blood, sometimes more, are found on your pants occurring between proper bleeds. A few women stop having periods at all. Far from being a problem, lack of bleeding usually goes hand-in-hand with better protection from pregnancy. This is because bleeding may stop when the progestogen-only pill has prevented ovulation from occurring.

You should note any unpleasant side effects and report them to your doctor. You may need to wait to see if these effects pass, or whether you should try a different pill.

Risks of the Progestogen-Only Pill

While using the progestogen-only pill, there is a slightly higher risk that if you do become pregnant it would be an ectopic pregnancy (i.e. inside the fallopian tube). However, this is a very rare event and is still less likely to happen than if you were using no contraception at all. You may also be more likely to suffer simple cysts, forming in the tissue left in the ovaries after ovulation. These fluid-filled swellings are not at all dangerous, although occasionally they can cause abdominal pain. They usually disappear on their own without treatment.

Pregnancy, Breastfeeding and the Progestogen-Only Pill

The progestogen-only pill has no effect on your ability to become pregnant once you stop taking it. Just as with the combined pill, however, you are advised to stop taking the Pill one month before you want to start a baby. This is just so that you can be sure of the date of your *last* natural period when your pregnancy begins.

Your developing baby will not be affected because you have been on the progestogen-only pill. Studies show that women who have become pregnant while taking it or immediately after stopping it are not more likely to suffer miscarriage, ectopic pregnancy or stillbirth or to have a baby with disabilities.

Neither do you have anything to worry about if you take the progestogen-only pill during the first few weeks, or even longer, of a pregnancy because you didn't realize you were pregnant. You should stop as soon as you know you are pregnant, but many studies have shown no increase in abnormalities or problems to babies born when this happens.

The progestogen-only pill does not affect breast milk, so it can be used while breastfeeding. What is more, the combination of breastfeeding and taking this pill gives almost 100 per cent protection from pregnancy. If you wanted to start or go back onto the progestogen-only pill having had your baby, you would start it 21 days after giving birth.

Injectables

Also known as the injection or the jab.

Injectable contraception is an injection of hormones that can prevent you getting pregnant for two to three months, depending on which injection you have. Injections of progestogen (synthetic progesterone) were first used in 1960 as a treatment for miscarriages and endometriosis, a condition where the tissue normally found lining the womb starts growing elsewhere in the body. As it was found to prevent ovulation, it was soon seen to be an effective method of birth control. At present, around 2.5 million women in 90 countries use injectables. However, in some, such as the USA, it is not licensed for contraceptive use yet.

Injectables are a very effective method of contraception. Fewer than one woman gets pregnant out of every hundred using this method over a year. It is worth noting, however, that

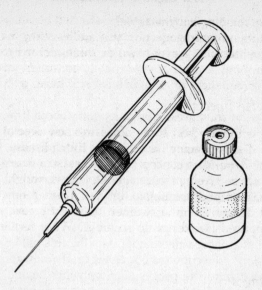

Figure 6: Injectable contraception

progestogen-only methods seem to be less effective in women weighing over 70 kg (11 stones), although this is more a problem for the progestogen-only pill and implants than for injectable methods.

Progestogen is injected deep into the muscles of your shoulder or buttocks. It dissolves very slowly, releasing a steady amount of the hormone into your body. There are two injectables used in the UK. The more common, Depo Provera, gives you 12 weeks' protection. The other, Noristerat, protects you for eight weeks. The injectable's main action is to stop an egg being released, and it also acts on the cervical mucus, making it form a sticky barrier to sperm. The lining of the womb would be thin and unwelcoming to any egg that *does* become fertilized. Progestogen also seems to act on the fallopian tubes, so they will not help sperm to travel up to meet an egg, nor any fertilized egg to travel down.

How Do You Use an Injectable?
Depending on which injection you are receiving, you visit a doctor or nurse once every two or three months to have an injection.

Can I Use Injectables?

Women who have had some illnesses such as stroke, severe arterial disease, acute or chronic liver disease or some hormone-dependent cancers (such as breast or ovarian cancer) should not be given an injectable. Being overweight may also make this method unsuitable for you. There seems to be no medical reason why a women who can use injectable contraception should not do so for all of her fertile life.

Advantages

Injectables are one of the most effective, yet reversible, methods of birth control. An injection is also probably the most private and convenient method. You can't lose or forget it, as long as you go back for follow-up injections, and no-one can tell you are using it. Injectables do not interfere with lovemaking. Many women say the injectable makes them feel well and that period pains are less. The unpleasant symptoms of PMS and menstruation are reduced by injectables.

Disadvantages

You do have to remember to visit your doctor every two or three months. Most women using the injectable find their periods are disturbed. Periods are likely to be irregular. They may initially be heavy or you might get light bleeding at any time, with no regular bleeds. As you continue using the method, bleeding can become less and less until you have no periods at all. This is not harmful. If you experience any side effects, they may persist until the injection wears off. And if you are afraid of injections themselves, this method could be unacceptable to you.

Side Effects
Some women using injectables, as with all progestogen contraception, may experience acne, greasy hair, dark skin patches, stomach cramps, bloating, headaches, dizzy spells, back pain, depression and mood changes, tiredness or loss of sexual interest. However, if you do experience any of these side effects, they are likely to be mild and short-lived. Periods are often irregular and may stop altogether, particularly after a second injection. This is not harmful to your health. Some women experience a degree of weight gain but this can vary. You may also find that when you want to have a baby your periods will take some time to return to normal and so there could be a delay in your getting pregnant.

Risks
There are no serious illnesses linked to using injectable contraception.

Pregnancy and Breastfeeding

You can only rely on each injection for two or three months, depending on which type you have been given. But it *can* take up to nine months or longer to become pregnant after stopping using this method. This is more likely if you have been using Depo Provera than Noristerat.

You are most unlikely to get pregnant while still on the injectable. Research suggests that becoming pregnant either while using this method or at any time after has no harmful effects on you or any child.

Injectables do not stop you breastfeeding your baby and seem to increase a woman's milk. Research shows that there are no harmful effects to a baby. However, injectables are not advised until six weeks after birth.

Implants

Implants are tiny, soft rods of silastic – a type of plastic – or hollow capsules, filled with the hormone progestogen (synthetic progesterone). Implants are put under the skin of a woman's inner upper arm, where they gradually release the hormone into the bloodstream. Implants are not yet available

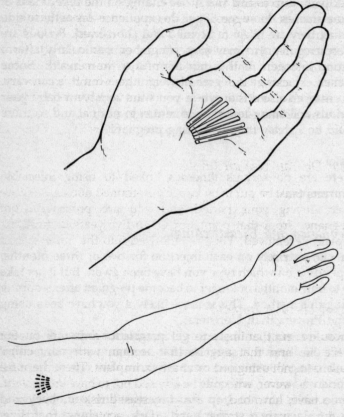

Figure 7: Implants

in the UK (they are already in use in the USA), but the one soon to be in use is Norplant, which consists of six of these rods, each measuring around 30 mm long and 2 mm wide.

The implant is one of the most effective contraceptive methods there is, and fewer than one woman in 100 will get pregnant while using it. This is probably because you can't lose, damage or forget to use your implant, as long as you go back for a further implant when one runs out. Implants are effective for up to five years, depending on the type you use. Some studies do suggest that the implant is less effective in women who weigh more than 70 kg (11 stones).

Implants mainly work by preventing ovulation. In addition, the progestogen in the implant makes the cervical mucus thicker, blocking the entrance of the womb to sperm. Progestogen also acts on the lining of the womb, making it thin and unwelcoming to any fertilized egg.

How Do You Use an Implant?

Implants must be put in by a specially-trained doctor. They are fitted during your period and you are protected from pregnancy from that point, for up to five years or until the implant is removed. They are inserted into the inner side of the upper arm.

Can I Use An Implant?

It would seem that implants are suitable for any stage of your fertile life and that any healthy woman with no medical reasons for not using one can have an implant. There are some women, however, who may be advised not to have an implant. If you have, have had, or are at increased risk of developing conditions such as stroke, heart attack, acute or chronic liver disease or hormone-dependent cancers (such as breast or ovarian cancer) you may be advised not to have an implant.

Advantages of the Implant

The method is extremely effective, long-lasting and safe. If you need a highly effective method but can't use the combined pill, which contains oestrogen, you could still have an implant. If you do suffer any unpleasant side effects, or want to become pregnant, one advantage of the implant is that the effect wears off very quickly after you have it removed. The implant doesn't interfere with lovemaking and, apart from regular checks with your doctor, needs no attention from you.

Disadvantages Of The Implant

The rods, although very small, may be seen under the skin in some women and they can be felt. So, unlike other methods of contraception, anyone knowing what they are may be able to see what method you are using. Most women using the implant find their periods are disturbed. You might get light bleeding at any time, with no regular bleeds. As you continue using the method, bleeding can become less and less until you have no periods at all. Since the method is still fairly new and not all doctors will have been trained to insert and remove implants, you may have to travel some distance to find one who can do so when it becomes available.

Side Effects
As with all progestogen-only methods, irregular periods tend to be the main difficulty with the implant, although bleeding is usually lighter. You may find this a problem, although knowing about it in advance could make it easier to cope with. Some women may have problems with weight gain, acne, greasy hair, stomach cramps, bloating, headaches, dizzy spells, back pain, depression and mood changes, tiredness or loss of sexual interest. If you do experience any of these, however, they are likely to be mild and short-lived, but do see your doctor or clinic if you are concerned. Some women may

find it uncomfortable to have the rods inserted, although a local anaesthetic is used. The procedure may also leave tiny scars, either when the rods are inserted or when they are removed.

Risks
There are no serious illnesses linked to using an implant.

Pregnancy and Breastfeeding

If you do want to get pregnant, you simply have the implants removed. There would be no effect on a baby if you got pregnant having had an implant removed. At present, we do not know if there would be any problems if you did become pregnant while using this method. But babies born to women using other progestogen contraception, such as the progestogen-only pill, have not been found to have problems. You can breastfeed at the same time as having an implant.

The Vaginal Ring

The vaginal ring is a soft, doughnut-shaped ring made of silastic – a type of plastic – which contains the hormone progestogen (synthetic progesterone). It is about the size of a small diaphragm. When left in the vagina, the ring slowly releases progestogen. In common with other progestogen-only contraceptive methods, the vaginal ring acts by altering cervical mucus, causing it to become sticky and so stopping sperm from entering the womb. The ring also prevents ovulation in some menstrual cycles.

The vaginal ring is slightly less effective than the progestogen-only pill, and studies so far suggest that four to five women out of every 100 using it for a year may fall pregnant. As with other progestogen-only methods, efficacy may be reduced in women weighing over 70 kilograms (11 stones).

The vaginal ring is not yet available in the UK. The one soon to be available will last for three months. There are currently other vaginal rings being developed which may last longer and there are also versions being developed that use both oestrogen and progestogen.

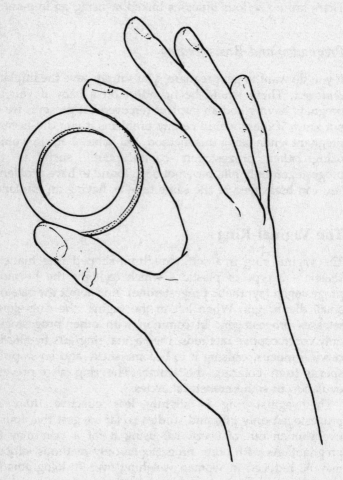

Figures 8a and b: The vaginal ring

How Do You Use a Vaginal Ring?

You squeeze the sides of the ring together to form a tampon shape and then slide the ring into your vagina. It can sit at any point in the vagina and is kept in place by muscles in the vaginal wall. You leave the ring inside the vagina all the time, including during your period and when you have sexual intercourse. You can use tampons with a vaginal ring in place. If the ring does come out for any reason, you simply put it back in again straight away. Every three months you take it out and replace it with a new one.

Future rings which release oestrogen as well as progestogen would be left in the vagina for three weeks and removed for one week, during which you would have a period.

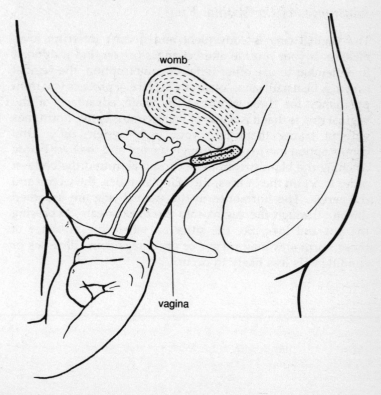

womb

vagina

Can I Use The Vaginal Ring?

If you have a prolapsed womb – when the womb slips down into the vagina – or don't have very good muscle tone in your vagina, you may not be able to keep the ring in place. If you don't like touching your vagina, using the ring might also be difficult. You may also find it difficult if you often suffer from constipation.

As far as studies show, you can use the vaginal ring for all of your fertile life. Women who have had pelvic inflammatory disease or an ectopic pregnancy or who have a vaginal or cervical infection will not be able to use a vaginal ring.

Advantages of the Vaginal Ring

The vaginal ring is convenient and doesn't interrupt love-making. If your routine often changes or you find it difficult to remember to use other types of contraception, the vaginal ring may be useful since, once put in place, it protects you from pregnancy for three months. The main advantage of the vaginal ring is that it is a way of using contraceptive hormones without taking them into your body system fully. Oral contraception has to pass through the gut and the liver before reaching the bloodstream to be carried all round the body in order to act on the ovaries, the fallopian tubes, the womb and the cervix. The hormones in the vaginal ring are absorbed directly through the vagina into the bloodstream, bypassing the gut and liver. So, the situation where the presence of these hormones may trigger or encourage some illnesses or conditions is less likely to occur.

Disadvantages of the Vaginal Ring

You may get irregular periods and have bleeding in between periods. Some women also get irritation in the vagina. You have to be aware when going to the loo while wearing a vaginal ring that if you push down too hard while having a motion or pulling out a tampon, the ring can come out. However, this is not a major disadvantage since all you have to do is put it back in place. If the ring has become soiled, it can be washed in clean water. The ring may become discoloured with use, but this does not affect the way it works.

Side Effects
A small number of women have reported irritation or a discharge when using the ring. As with all progestogen methods of contraception, you may also find periods becoming irregular and you could have 'spotting' in between periods.

Risks
As with the progestogen-only pill, there is a slightly higher risk that if you do become pregnant it would be an ectopic pregnancy – where an egg lodges in and starts to grow in a fallopian tube instead of in the womb. However, this is a very rare event. You are more likely to have it happen if you were using no contraception at all. You may also be more likely to suffer ovarian cysts, forming in the tissue left in the ovaries after ovulation. These fluid-filled swellings are not at all dangerous, although occasionally they can cause abdominal pain. They usually disappear on their own without treatment.

Pregnancy and Breastfeeding

If you want to get pregnant, you simply remove the ring. Research on other progestogen-only methods suggests that there are no abnormalities or problems in babies born to mothers becoming pregnant after using them. If you became pregnant while using a ring, you should remove it, but leaving the ring in for a time because you didn't realize you were pregnant is not thought to harm a baby. After pregnancy, your doctor or clinic will advise you when you can restart this method.

CHAPTER THREE

Barrier Methods

Barrier methods prevent pregnancy by stopping the meeting of egg and sperm. An additional advantage of these methods is that condoms, diaphragms and caps prevent more than pregnancy. They can also protect against a range of illnesses and infections. Women using them have less cancer of the cervix or pre-cancerous changes and some sexually transmitted infections than women using other methods of birth control.

The Male Condom

Also known as sheath, johnnie, French letter, rubber.

A male condom is a thin, latex rubber tube that is closed at one end. It is designed to cover the penis during lovemaking and to catch the man's sperm after he climaxes so that it cannot get into his partner's vagina. Male condoms can be simple tubes or be shaped to fit more snugly behind the glans (head of the penis). They now come in a range of colours and may have ribbing or bumps on them. Some are scented or flavoured. Most male condoms are lubricated, to make sex more comfortable. In many cases this lubrication is a spermicide (see page 75). Male condoms can be plain-ended or have a teat end, designed to make it easy to leave space at the end to contain semen.

Male condoms are hardly new. Some cave paintings and Egyptian murals appear to show men with some sort of covering over the penis. We don't know whether this was for sexual use – as birth control or protection from disease – or for decoration. (Some tribes today still use hollow reeds or sticks as penis covers to protect against insect bites and other injuries, and simply because it looks good.) Or these coverings could have been for some ritual purpose we don't understand. However, we *do* know that male condoms have been around for a long time. Early male condoms were made from sheep gut, linen, oiled silk or even leather. Technical developments in rubber manufacturing in the 1840s and in latex in the early 1930s made the modern male condom a possibility.

Male condoms are a popular form of contraception in many parts of the world. Some 40 million couples use them worldwide, but they are more popular in some countries than in others. Almost three-quarters of all couples using contraeption in Japan, for instance, rely on male condoms. The atest available figures show that 1.6 million women in the UK (around 1 in 8 couples) use male condoms as their main method of contraception, and just under 1 in 5 couples in the USA. Male condom use is going up as we become more aware of sexually transmitted diseases including HIV/AIDS.

Male condoms work as a barrier, stopping sperm and egg meeting. How well the condom protects you from pregnancy depends on how well you use it. The male condom *can* give you 98 per cent protection. But failure rates range between two and 15 couples out of every 100 having a pregnancy. The higher figures reflect pregnancies that are due to 'user failure'. That is, making a mistake with how you put on or take off the male condom, or having close genital touching before putting on or after taking off a male condom, so allowing it to be less of a protection.

Male condoms are available over the counter at various outlets. If you go to a clinic, you will be asked to give your name and address, but this is simply for clinic statistics. Nobody is 'checking up' on you. You may be offered a chance to talk to a doctor, nurse or counsellor, and this could be worthwhile. Remember, when people *do* get pregnant using the male condom it's often because mistakes were made in correct use. The doctor or nurse could help you practise (on

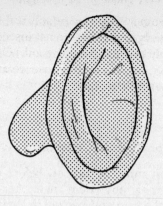

Figures 9a and b: The male condom

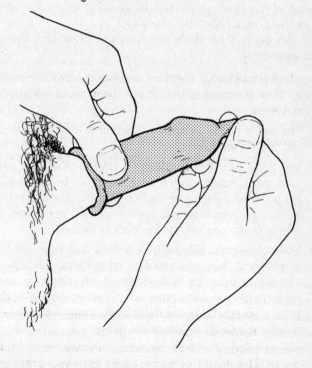

a plastic model or your finger, not the real thing!) so that you could feel confident about using this method. Visiting a clinic has two additional benefits. Firstly, male condoms are free on the NHS. Secondly, it gives both men and women the chance to have well person health care.

How Do You Use a Male Condom?

The male condom must be put on before the man's penis touches his partner anywhere near her genitals. Male condoms come rolled up and packed in their own individual foil or plastic wrapping. The idea is for you to slip one over the end of the erect penis and to unroll it down the shaft – like putting on a rolled-up stocking.

You can make your male condom use more effective with some easy tips:

1 Choose a brand of condom that has the BSI Kitemark on it. This guarantees that it has been made to specified standards.

2 The penis has to be firmly erect, or it may be difficult to roll the condom on.

3 You need to put a condom on *before* letting any part of your penis/vagina touch each other, or before touching his penis and then her vagina with the same hand. This is because you can get sperm in the 'pre-come' fluid which leaks out when the man is excited.

4 Male condoms, although very thin and fine, are tough and strong, but you need to treat them carefully. You shouldn't snag or scrape them on rings or ragged fingernails or poke them too hard when unrolling them. In fact, you should treat them in the same way you would handle a pair of tights or stockings.

5 When putting a male condom on, you should leave enough space in the tip to collect the semen. To get any

air out of the teat or closed end, you squeeze the condom tip shut as you slip it on to the end of the penis. If you don't, when he comes semen may push up the shaft and ooze out of the open end of the condom. It could then get into the vagina.

6 It's important for the man to pull out of the woman's vagina before he completely loses his erection soon after he has come, and to make sure the condom remains *on* as he does so. If you lie together after climax, his erection can soften and the male condom can slip off. When he pulls out, semen can then spill out and lead to a pregnancy. Either of you can put a finger or two on the condom at the base of his penis as he pulls out, to make sure the condom stays in place.

7 Use a new condom each time you make love.

The best way to use a male condom is to practise first. You can make it part of your lovemaking instead of an interruption. Men can practise putting one on themselves, and women can use a banana, a small cucumber or a deodorant bottle to get the feel of how to do it.

Putting on two male condoms at the same time, one over the other, does *not* make you twice as safe. Far from offering extra protection, the two layers rub against each other and wearing two can *increase* the chances of a condom breaking.

Male condoms do last for some time if the individual packet is unbroken. You will find a 'best used by' date stamped on the packet. However, if you keep them in a hot room or near a fire for long periods of time, they will perish much more quickly. Look also for the BSI 'Kitemark' on the packet that shows the condom was made by a reputable company and tested to high standards. Don't wash and re-use a male condom. They are strong, but may perish with this treatment. And never use oil or an oil-based cream for lubrication if you are using a male condom. This would include massage oil or bath oil, and any massage or face, hand or body moisturizing cream that contains oil. It would also include some medical products, such as pessaries, that might be prescribed for you by a doctor. Most products now have a full list of ingredients on them, so check and ask your pharmacist or doctor if you are not sure. Oil destroys the latex rubber of the male condom at an astonishing speed – within seconds. If you do want extra lubrication, use water-based lubricating jelly, such as KY Jelly, or a spermicidal cream. Once you have used a condom, throw it away carefully. Don't flush it down the toilet, but put it in a bin. You can wrap it in some tissue first if you want.

Can I Use Male Condoms?

Men who cannot have or keep a strong erection are likely to find the male condom unsuitable for them. If either partner gets a reaction from the spermicide or lubricant used on condoms they may want to try another type of condom without spermicide or lubricant. Religious taboos may make using a male condom difficult if you are not supposed to touch your genitals with both hands. You can get round this, of course, by helping each other. Physical disability may also make male condom use difficult if both partners have problems with holding and handling small objects.

You can use male condoms throughout your life, from first sex right through to the end of your life. Unlike most other forms of contraception, they can be useful for protection against sexual infections even when you don't need them to protect against pregnancy.

Advantages

The male condom is the only reversible male method of contraception. The male condom protects against more than pregnancy. Male condoms, when used properly, protect against most sexual infections, including chlamydia, non-specific urethritis (NSU), gonorrhoea, genital warts, herpes and pelvic inflammatory disease (PID). PID is when sexual infection passes to the reproductive areas of the female body such as the womb, the fallopian tubes and the walls of the pelvic cavity. PID causes inflammation which leads to scarring, and scar tissue can often build up, to bind together your tubes and ovaries. In the worse cases this can lead to infertility. Most important of all, male condoms can protect both partners from contracting HIV, the virus that can lead to AIDS. Women who start having sex while in their early teens and have more than one sexual partner have an increased risk of developing cancer of the cervix, and using a male condom can help protect against this.

Male condoms are also fun to use. There are plenty of different types – different shapes, different textures, different colours and now different scents and flavours. They are also easy to get. If sex is a spur-of-the-moment thing, you can usually find a garage, bar or late-night shop which sells them. Or you can buy them with your usual shopping without having to see a doctor. Condoms are also very useful if you don't want to feel wet after having sex. If you would rather go straight to sleep, or you want to go out immediately afterwards, or even if you want to make love outdoors, using a condom can catch the semen and keep the woman relatively dry.

Male condoms may also help if his climax comes too quickly. Although today's male condoms are very thin and sensitive and don't 'spoil' lovemaking, for some people they can slow you down just a little bit – enough to be helpful at times.

Another advantage of a male condom is that you know you have used it and can see at once if anything has gone wrong. If it has, you can then see a doctor immediately to discuss emergency contraception (see page 113). It is a particularly useful method if you don't make love very often and don't want to use a method that gives protection every day, such as the Pill or an IUD.

Disadvantages

For it to work, you have to use a male condom properly every time you make love. You do have to think ahead of time and to recognize you are likely to have sex and make sure you have a condom handy. You have to feel comfortable about touching yourself or your partner intimately and not to be worried about the image of the male condom having to do with 'dirty' or promiscuous sex.

Side Effects
For most users, there are no side effects from the male condom itself. Some people can have a sensitivity to latex rubber, but this is extremely uncommon. Some men and women have found the lubricants or spermicides used can irritate. If your penis or vagina becomes red, sore or swollen because of this, you could alternate between spermicidally lubricated, lubricated or unlubricated male condoms to find one that feels comfortable. In the UK, there are special non-allergy-causing male condoms which do not use a spermicide and use lubrication that does not cause allergic reactions.

Risks
None.

Pregnancy and Breastfeeding

If you want to get pregnant, you simply stop using the male condom. Using a male condom before getting pregnant, or getting pregnant while using one, can have no possible harmful effect on a baby. Male condoms can, however, protect mother and father against catching a sexual infection that otherwise might have harmed all three. A male condom is an excellent method to use while breastfeeding as it can have no harmful effects on the health of mother or child.

The Female Condom

The female condom would seem to be a new method of contraception. However, some 2nd century writing suggests slipping the bladder of a goat into your partner's vagina to protect her from the harmful effects of semen. And pictures of Casanova blowing up sheaths suggest that loose-fitting male condoms may once have functioned as do today's female variety. In the 1920s, Marie Stopes, the birth control pioneer, advocated the use of a rubber female condom.

The female condom is a loose tube designed to line the vagina. It protects the vagina and vulva from contact with body fluids from the male, and acts as a barrier, stopping a meeting between sperm and egg. There is one female condom presently available in the UK, called Femidom. This is made of soft polyurethane, has a ring around its open end, and a loose ring that lies inside the closed end. This loose ring is folded and guided inside the vagina, past the pubic bone. This ring helps the female condom to stay in place, lining the vagina. The open end of the condom lies flat against the vulva. Other female condoms, of a similar or different design, made of polyurethane or latex, will be available in the near future. One such, the bikini condom, is described in chapter 10.

Female condoms are available over the counter at various outlets. Some clinics do offer them. If you go to a clinic, you may be offered a chance to talk to a doctor, nurse or counsellor, and this could be worthwhile. The doctor or nurse could help you practise putting the female condom in place, so that you could feel confident about using this method. Visiting a clinic has two additional benefits. Firstly, supplies are free on the NHS. Secondly, it would give you the chance to have well woman health care.

How Do You Use A Female Condom?

The female condom is put inside the vagina before there is any genital contact. As with the male condom, you have to take reasonable care not to snag it on rings or sharp fingernails. You would also have to take care that the female condom is not pushed up too far into the vagina. If this happens, the penis can slip outside the female condom and the protective effect is lost. How well the female condom protects you from pregnancy could depends on how well you use it. It is

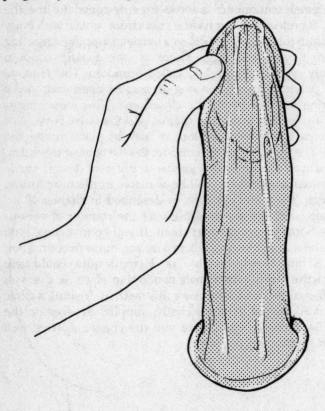

Figures 10a and b: The female condom

estimated that female condoms will be as effective as male condoms when used correctly.

You can make your condom use more effective with some easy tips:

1 You can put a female condom in any time before making love.

2 You need to put a condom in *before* letting any part of your penis/vagina touch each other, or before touching his penis and then her vagina with the same hand. This is because you can get sperm in the 'pre-come' fluid which leaks out when the man is aroused.

3 Female condoms are thin but tough and strong; however, you need to treat them carefully. You shouldn't snag or scrape them on rings or ragged fingernails.

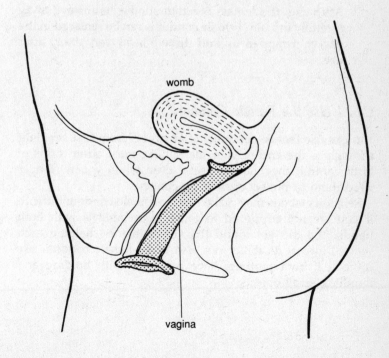

4 Use a new female condom each time you have sex. Don't wash and re-use a female condom. They are strong, but may perish with this treatment.

5 Unlike the male condom, which is made of latex, a female condom made of polyurethane will not perish if it comes into contact with oil or an oil-based cream. This means you can use any massage oil or cream you like in your sex play, and you also don't have to worry about creams or pessaries prescribed by your doctor for use in the vagina or rectum having any harmful effects. You can use lubricating jelly or a spermicidal cream as well, but you don't need to use spermicides to give you extra protection.

6 To remove the female condom, you simply twist the end to prevent semen spilling and gently pull it out.

7 After use, the female condom should be thrown away carefully in a bin. Female condoms can be replaced in the packet, wrapped up and thrown away very easily after use.

Can I Use the Female Condom?

You can use female condoms at any time, from first sex right through to the end of your life. Unlike most other forms of birth control, they can be useful even when you no longer need them to protect against pregnancy.

Religious taboos may make using a female condom difficult if you are not supposed to touch your genitals with both hands. You can get round this, of course, by helping each other. Physical disability can also make female condom use difficult if both partners have problems with holding and handling small objects.

Advantages

The female condom protects against more than pregnancy. Female condoms protect against most sexual infections including non-specific urethritis (NSU), gonorrhoea, genital warts, herpes and pelvic inflammatory disease (PID). PID is when sexual infection passes to the reproductive areas of your body such as the womb, the fallopian tubes and the walls of the pelvic cavity. PID causes inflammation which leads to scarring, and scar tissue can often build up, to bind together your tubes and ovaries. In the worse cases this can lead to infertility. Most important of all, it can protect both partners from contracting HIV, the virus that can lead to AIDS. Women who start having sex while in their early teens or who have several sexual partners have an increased risk of developing cancer of the cervix, and using a female condom can protect against this. It gives women the high degree of protection also offered by the male condom, but in their own hands. An additional advantage in using the female condom is that the man does not have to pull out as soon as he has come. The couple can lie together without worrying that losing his erection may result in the condom becoming displaced and releasing semen into the vagina, as it would with the male condom. It can also be used when the man finds it difficult to have a full erection.

Female condoms are available over the counter and you don't have to see a doctor in order to get them. As with male condoms, female condoms are also very useful if you don't want to feel wet after having sex. If you would rather go straight to sleep or you want to go out immediately afterwards, or even if you want to make love outdoors, using a female condom can catch the semen and keep the woman relatively dry.

Another advantage female condoms share with male condoms is that you know you have used it and can see at once if anything has gone wrong. You can then see a doctor immediately to discuss emergency contraception (see page 113). It is a particularly useful method if you don't make love very often and don't want to use a method that gives protection every day, such as the Pill or an IUD.

Disadvantages

For it to be effective, you have to use a female condom properly every time you make love. You do have to think ahead of time and to recognize you are likely to have sex and make sure you have a female condom handy. You have to be comfortable about touching yourself intimately. Some people don't like the way the female condom shows outside the vagina. You do have to use the female condom with care, and women with poor vaginal muscle tone may not be able to use it.

Side Effects
There are no side effects from the female condom itself.

Risks
None.

Pregnancy and Breastfeeding

If you want to get pregnant, simply stop using the female condom. Using a female condom before getting pregnant, or becoming pregnant while using a female condom, can have no possible harmful effect on a baby. Female condoms can, however, protect mother and father against catching a sexual infection that otherwise might have harmed all three.

A female condom is an excellent method to use while breastfeeding, as it can have no harmful effects on the health of mother or child.

Diaphragms And Caps

Also known as 'Dutch caps' or 'the cap'.

Diaphragms and caps may be some of the oldest forms of birth control. The women of Sumatra used to mould opium resin into a cup shaped to fit over the cervix, and Hungarian women used beeswax in the same way. The Romans used plugs of wool soaked in gum, and 18th-century French women used the squeezed half of a lemon.

A diaphragm or a cap acts as a barrier, preventing sperm reaching the cervix and travelling through to the womb. They will also hold a spermicide (see page 75) in place, to kill sperm. Although the names 'diaphragm' and 'cap' are often used to mean the same thing, they are actually two different devices. The diaphragm is the more commonly used of the two.

Diaphragms, also known as Dutch caps, are soft latex domes with a flexible metal rim. There are three types, all of which come in different sizes. They measure from 55 mm to 100 mm across, going up in 5 mm stages. The Flat Spring has a rim which contains a firm, flat metal band. They measure from 55 to 95 mm across. The Coil Spring has a rim which contains a spiral of coiled wire. They come in sizes from 55 mm to 100 mm. The Arcing Spring has a rim which combines the features of the other two and these come in sizes of 60 mm to 95 mm.

Cervical caps are made entirely from rubber and are smaller than diaphragms. There are also three types of these. The Cervical Cap or Prentif Cavity Rim is shaped like a thimble, with a thick rim and a deep, soft top. It comes in four sizes ranging from 23 mm to 31 mm, going up in 3 mm stages. The Vault or Dumas Cap is a shallow, semi-circular dome which comes in five sizes from 55 mm to 75 mm. The Vimule Cap is a combination of the Vault and Cervical Cap. It is dome-shaped with a thin rim and comes in three sizes from 45 mm to 51 mm.

Between 10 and 11 per cent of couples all over the world use this sort of barrier method. In the UK, two per cent of users – around 200,000 women – use diaphragms or caps.

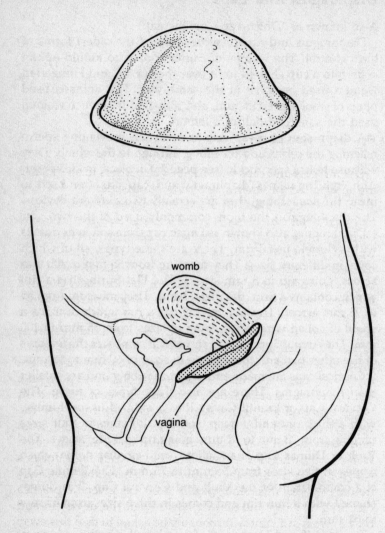

Figures 11a and b: The diaphragm

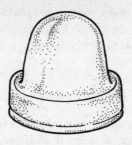

Figure 12: The cervical cap

Diaphragms and caps work mainly as barriers to sperm and are more effective when used with spermicide.

Studies suggest that out of every hundred women using a diaphragm or cap correctly over a year, two to three will become pregnant. Other studies suggest from two to 15 women. The more carefully and correctly the guidelines for using these methods are followed, the more effective they will be. Some studies have been carried out to check how effective it would be to use a diaphragm without spermicides. Many women would prefer this option. The conclusion at present is that you should *always* use spermicides with a diaphragm or cap to give you maximum effectiveness for these methods.

You don't need a full medical check-up to get a diaphragm or cap, although you might welcome the chance to have one. But you will need an internal examination to see if this method is right for you and to measure you for size. If you use the wrong type and size for you it won't protect you from pregnancy, and it may cause discomfort and cystitis in some women. You may be seen by a nurse at your own doctor's surgery or at a clinic, as many nurses have the necessary training to do this. You would then be given a practice diaphragm or cap and shown how to put the device in and how to get it out. You will probably be asked to take this away and practise putting it in and taking it out. You would be advised not to rely on it yet for contraception and be asked to return to your next appointment with the diaphragm or cap in place. If there have been no problems and you feel confident, you will be given your diaphragm or cap and a supply of spermicides.

How Do You Use a Diaphragm Or Cap?

You can put a diaphragm or cap into the vagina any time before having sex. However, if more than three hours have passed between putting it in and having intercourse, you will need to add more spermicide. You can also put it in as part of sex play, as long as you don't have close genital contact before that.

Diaphragm

If you are using a diaphragm, you squeeze some spermicide cream or jelly on both sides of the dome and a tiny amount on the rim. Alternatively, you could use spermicidal foam or film.

The rim of the diaphragm is then pinched together so that it can be inserted into the vagina. Flat Spring diaphragms fold into a flat shape, while Coil Spring diaphragms are more flexible. Both are similar in size and shape to a tampon when squeezed in this way. Arcing Spring diaphragms form an arc like a small banana. When guided up towards the top of the vagina, the diaphragm opens out to cover the cervix. Either partner can do this and check with a finger to see that the diaphragm is properly in place. It should cover the cervix entirely and stay behind the pubic bone, which can be felt just inside the vagina entrance, behind the upper wall. If more than three hours pass before you have sex, you would need to put in some more spermicide without removing the diaphragm. You can use any form of spermicide – pessaries, film, foam or cream or jelly using an applicator (see page 75). And if you have sex more than once, add some more spermicide, too.

The diaphragm should be left in place for at least six hours after your last lovemaking, to allow the spermicide to continue working. Rather than have a bath during this time, it would be better to wash or take a shower, as a bath in some cases may wash out the spermicide without removing all the sperm. If your period starts while a diaphragm is in place, it will simply collect the blood. This won't harm you in any way. But you shouldn't leave a diaphragm, or any barrier method, inside you for more than 30 hours.

You remove a diaphragm by passing your index finger into your vagina, hooking the rim of the diaphragm and pulling it out.

Cap

If you are using one of the smaller caps, you put spermicide only on the inside, but not on the rim. You then insert the cap into the vagina so that the open end fits snugly over the cervix. These caps are held in place by suction. Once the cap is in place, more spermicide is added.

You remove a cap by hooking or knocking the rim of the cap off the cervix. This releases the suction which holds the cap in place and it can then be pulled out. If you have any difficulty, bear down as if you were passing a motion. This will push the cervix down within easier reach.

After removing the diaphragm or cap, wash it in warm water with plain unscented soap, dry it and then store it safely in a container in a cool place. You should check your diaphragm or cap each time you wash it, for holes or thin spots. To do this, hold the diaphragm or cap up to the light and look carefully. Never let any oil-based creams or lubricants touch it. This includes body or bath oils, or any moisturizing creams that could contain oil, or petroleum jellies such as Vaseline. This also includes any pessaries or creams for genital or anal use which a doctor or a pharmacist has given you. If you are using a diaphragm or cap you should see a doctor or nurse for a check every six to twelve months. You would need to get a new diaphragm or cap at least every two years, and if you have a baby, a miscarriage or an abortion, or if you gain or lose more than 3 kg, you should see your doctor or nurse to check if you need another size. You don't need to worry, however, if your diaphragm discolours or the rim becomes slightly misshapen. You can gently ease it back into shape. If you do have any worries, get it checked by a nurse or doctor.

Can I Use a Diaphragm or Cap?

Diaphragms or caps can be used at any time in your fertile life, except for the six weeks following childbirth. However, you may find your own body, personal taste, your lifestyle or your culture could make it difficult for you to use these methods. If you have short fingers or a long vagina, often suffer urinary infections or have had toxic shock syndrome, the diaphragm or cap may be unsuitable for you. If the muscles in your vagina are loose, or you have a prolapse (where the womb slumps down into the vagina) or if your womb is retroverted (tilted back), you may have less choice. An Arcing Spring diaphragm can be used in this situation, but you may not be able to keep other diaphragms, or caps, in place.

Anyone who finds it difficult or unpleasant to touch themselves would find this an unsatisfactory method of contraception. They would also be difficult to use if you had little privacy and couldn't get to a bathroom easily. It's not a good method if animals or children in your home are liable to get hold of it and chew it or use it as a frisbee! Also, couples from a culture that forbids men and women to touch themselves intimately with one of their hands may find this not a method of choice – unless they are happy to help each other. People with physical disability or other special needs may also find this is not a method of choice, or is one that needs co-operation between partners.

Advantages

Diaphragms and cap have no harmful effects on health. They can protect the cervix against some sexual infections and against diseases such as cancer of the cervix and pelvic inflammatory disease (PID). PID is when sexual infection passes to the reproductive areas of your body such as the womb, the fallopian tubes and the walls of the pelvic cavity. PID causes inflammation which leads to scarring, and scar tissue can often build up, to bind together your tubes and ovaries. In the worst cases this can lead to infertility.

Diaphragms and caps are easy to use and are only needed when you actually make love, although you can put them in at any time prior to sex. They are also a barrier method that is in the woman's control. Once you have your device it will last for up to two years, as long as it is used and looked after carefully. Of course, you will need to have six- to twelve-monthly checks to make sure all is well.

Disadvantages

You have to put your diaphragm or cap in every time you make love, you must use care when using it and some can find it fiddly and messy. Men may feel the device during intercourse. You do need to see a trained medical person to find out the correct type and size of diaphragm or cap for you. Diaphragms and caps can be uncomfortable to either partner if the device does not fit properly. The firm rim of a diaphragm can put pressure on your bladder, through the thin walls of the vagina, especially if it is the wrong size. You may then develop cystitis, an infection in the bladder or water passage. If this does happen, you should see your doctor or nurse to have the size and fit checked. If the problem remains, change to a small, rimless cap. Some people may also experience irritation from spermicides.

Side Effects
There are no harmful side effects to using a diaphragm or cap correctly.

Risks
There is a small risk from toxic shock syndrome. This is caused by bacteria that can enter into the bloodstream through tiny breaks in the skin of the vagina. It is more likely to happen if anything – a tampon or a diaphragm or cap – is left in the vagina for long periods. This is why it is not recommended to leave a diaphragm or cap in place for longer than 30 hours at the most.

Pregnancy and Breastfeeding

If you want to get pregnant, simply stop using the method. If you've used a diaphragm or cap, with or without spermicides, in the past before getting pregnant, there will be no effect on a pregnancy or a baby. If you do get pregnant while using them, there will be no harmful effects, either.

You can use a diaphragm or cap while breastfeeding. However, you would have to wait for six weeks after giving birth, or until your vagina has regained its muscle tone. And you would need to see your doctor or nurse to have a check, as you may need a new size.

CHAPTER FOUR

Chemical Methods

Spermicides

Spermicides are chemicals which prevent pregnancy by killing sperm. These chemicals come as creams and jellies, squares of film, foam or pessaries (small, solid pieces of cream). Spermicides may be the most ancient, original form of birth control. As long ago as 2,000 BC, women were putting sticky mixtures of honey, gum arabic and crocodile dung in themselves, to block and slow down sperm.

Around one per cent – about 100,000 – of women in the UK rely on spermicides as a single method of contraception. Many more use them with caps, diaphragms and condoms and make use of them in the sponge.

Spermicides work in two ways. Firstly, the chemicals in the spermicides have an effect on the sperm. Sperm needs to be lively and strong to be able to swim up through the entrance to the womb and to then reach the fallopian tubes and any awaiting egg. The spermicidal chemicals rob sperm of that ability to swim, so that they come to a halt and cannot continue their journey and die. The active ingredient in most UK spermicides is Nonoxynol 9, which may also give some protection from many sexually transmitted infections, including HIV, the virus that can lead to AIDS. Secondly, they act as a barrier. The melting film or pessary or the mass of foam, cream or jelly pools around the entrance to the womb and stops any surviving sperm entering.

Spermicides are *not* an effective method to use on their own. Between four and 25 women out of every hundred using spermicides on their own for a year would become pregnant.

Spermicides, as with all methods, are most effective if you use them every time you make love and follow the instructions carefully. They are also more effective if you use sexual positions other than woman-on-top or standing up (these allow spermicide to trickle out of you). The interval between inserting a spermicide and making love is also important. It needs to be long enough for the chemicals to have started to work, but not too long, or the chemicals become inactive. The instructions that come with each product will tell you how long to leave.

Some spermicides are better on their own than others. Jellies, films and creams are excellent when used with condoms or diaphragms or caps, but foam is best if you are *only* going to use a spermicide. This is because foams spread better in the vagina, forming a more effective barrier. The bubbles in the foam also trap sperm, giving the spermicide longer to kill them. Foam is effective immediately.

Spermicides are available over the counter at various outlets. If you go to a clinic, you may be offered a chance to talk to a

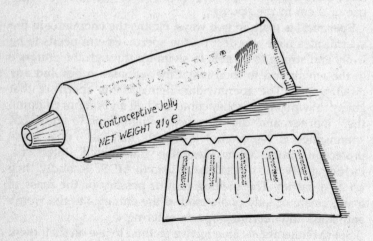

Figure 13: Spermicidal jelly and pessaries

doctor, nurse or counsellor, and this could be worthwhile, so that you could feel confident about using this method. Visiting a clinic has two additional benefits. Firstly, supplies are free on the NHS. Secondly, it would give both men and women the chance to have well person health care.

How Do You Use Spermicides?

Spermicides need to be placed high up in the vagina, around the entrance to the womb. A pessary or a square of film can be pushed into place with a finger and then left for three to 10 minutes to dissolve. Creams, jellies or film can be put inside the bowl of a cap or diaphragm and smoothed onto the outside of a diaphragm. Foams or creams can be inserted gently inside the vagina using an applicator. Applicators are like a tampon applicator or a syringe without a needle.

If you have intercourse more than once, you would need to add more spermicide. And if you delay having intercourse for more than three hours after putting in a spermicide, you would need to insert some more. You must also be careful not to wash out your vagina for six hours after having sex.

Can I Use Spermicides?

You can use spermicides as a method of contraception at any time throughout your fertile life, and as protection from infection at any time. Some people do find the chemicals or any perfume used in the spermicides cause irritation. If it is particularly important that you don't become pregnant, relying solely on spermicides for birth control would not be an ideal choice.

Advantages of Spermicides

There are no health risks. You don't have to use the method every day, only at the times when you make love. Spermicides are available over the counter and you don't have to see a doctor to get them. You are less likely to suffer some sexually transmitted infections if you are using spermicides. Spermicides can also make lovemaking more comfortable by adding extra lubrication to the vagina.

Disadvantages of Spermicides

Spermicides are best used as an addition to a barrier method such as condom, cap or diaphragm. They are not very effective on their own. And they can make sex *too* slippery so that both of you can lose sensation.

Side Effects
Side effects with spermicides are uncommon, but some people react to them, developing redness, irritation and soreness in the vagina or outside on the vulva, or on the penis. If this happens to you, stop using the spermicide and see a doctor for advice.

Risks
None.

Pregnancy and Breastfeeding

If you want to become pregnant, you simply stop using the method.

A baby will not be affected by your having used spermicides in the past, and spermicides do not affect breastfeeding.

The Sponge

The sponge is made of soft polyurethane soaked in a spermicide. It is shaped like a button mushroom with a dimple on one side, and measures 5.5 cm across and 2.5 cm thick. For centuries, women have been using natural sponges, wads of material and even moss or the pith of reeds to soak up both menstrual blood and semen. Our ancestors would have dipped the sponge or cotton wool into lemon, vinegar, wine, crocodile dung, gum arabic or honey. These either formed a plug as a barrier against sperm, or made the vagina too acidic for the sperm to be able to move.

The main action of the sponge is to be a carrier for spermicide. It also can cover the cervix and act as a barrier to sperm. The sponge is not a very effective form of contraception. Between nine and 25 women may get pregnant out of every 100 using it for a year.

Sponges are available over the counter at various outlets. Some clinics do supply them and you may be offered a chance to talk to a doctor, nurse or counsellor, and this could be worthwhile. The doctor or nurse could help you practise putting in the sponge so that you could feel confident about using this method. Visiting a clinic for over-the-counter contraception has two additional benefits. Firstly, it is then free on the NHS. Secondly, it would give you the chance to have well woman health care.

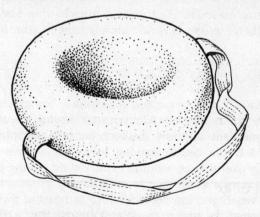

Figure 14: The contraceptive sponge

How Do You Use the Sponge?

You moisten the sponge with a small amount of water to activate the spermicide. The sponge will swell slightly and foam will appear as you squeeze it. You then push the sponge high into the vagina so that the dimple fits snugly over the cervix. You can put the sponge in place and forget about it for as long as 24 hours before having sex. You can also make love as many times as you like in that time without needing to add further spermicide. You leave the sponge in place for six hours after the last lovemaking and then pull it out by the loop of material attached and throw it away carefully. Don't throw it down the toilet, as you may find it floats and will not flush away. The sponge should not be left in place for more than 30 hours, and once removed, should *not* be reused. The sponge should also not be used during your period.

Can I Use the Sponge?

You should not use the sponge if you have any problems with cervical or vaginal infections. Using the sponge could be difficult if you have short fingers or a long vagina or a dislike of touching yourself. Poor vaginal muscle tone may make it more difficult to use. It is safe for any time in your fertile life.

Advantages of the Sponge

The method is easy to get and easy to use. You can make love as many times as you like without having to add more spermicide. It is also very discreet, because you can insert it up to 24 hours before making love. The sponge may be especially useful if you wouldn't really mind getting pregnant, or if you have a lesser chance of becoming pregnant anyway, such as when you are breastfeeding or nearing menopause.

The sponge is easier to insert and remove than a diaphragm or cap. The sponge is likely to offer some protection against sexual infections and cancer of the cervix, although not as much as condoms.

Disadvantages

The sponge is not as effective as many other methods of birth control and has a high pregnancy rate. Some women find the sponge uncomfortable. Some men can feel it while making love.

Side Effects
The spermicides in the sponge can cause irritation of the vagina, vulva or penis in a very few people.

Risks
None.

Pregnancy and Breastfeeding

If you want to become pregnant, simply stop using the method. A baby will not be affected by your having used a sponge in the past, and using the sponge has no effect on breastfeeding.

CHAPTER FIVE

The Intrauterine Device

Also known as the IUD.

Intrauterine devices (IUDs) are devices that are put in a woman's womb to prevent pregnancy. IUDs are hardly new. Desert tribes were said to put pebbles into the wombs of their camels to prevent the animals getting pregnant and so slowing them down on long journeys. In the last century, and early in this century, loops of catgut, silkworm gut or silver were recommended by various doctors in Germany. The most famous of these doctors was Grafenberg, who gave his name to the Grafenberg Ring. The method became unpopular in the 1930s and 1940s because of reports of medical complications.

When polyethylene was developed, the IUD became a useful and acceptable device again. This plastic has a 'memory', so that you can make a device in various shapes, such as a T or an upside-down U, which can be straightened out to insert it through the cervix into the womb. Once in place there, the device springs back into its original shape.

There have been several generations of modern IUDs. The first were made of plastic only, such as Lippes Loop and the Saf-T-Coil. The second generation were made of plastic and copper, such as the Gravigard Cu 7. The current, third, generation of IUDs, such as Novagard, are of various shapes and are made of polyethylene and copper wire, or copper wire with a silver core. They have two threads at one end. When the device is in place in the womb, these threads pass out through the cervical canal and hang down a short way into the vagina. These devices seem to stay in place better, produce lighter periods and less pain than the first generation plastic-only types. Their smaller size also makes them easier and less uncomfortable to put in. There are also hormonal IUDs. These are impregnated with slowly-releasing progestogen. These may soon be available in the UK.

Around seven per cent of women – some 900,000 – using contraception in the UK have an IUD. In some countries this device is even more popular. One in four women in Scandinavia and half the women in China using birth control choose the IUD as their method.

The IUD works in several ways. Having an object in the womb sets up various reactions in the body. The main action is through the copper released by the IUD which makes sperm slow down and an egg take longer over its journey through the fallopian tube, preventing fertilization. It is also likely that the lining of the womb becomes unwelcoming to any egg that does get fertilized, preventing it implanting and starting to develop.

Between one and three women out of every 100 get pregnant using the IUD. Most pregnancies happen in the first six months of IUD use, and the longer you use the method the less likely you are to become pregnant. The newer devices have even lower pregnancy rates.

The device must be inserted by a doctor, preferably one who has had specific training. *When* you have an IUD put in may be important. It has been found that it's easier and hurts less if the device is put in towards the end of a period. This is because the cervix is softer and more open at this stage of your monthly cycle. There is less chance of the IUD being pushed out by the normal contractions of the womb, which are stronger during heavy bleeding. Also, putting the device in place during a period is a guarantee that you are not pregnant at the time. IUDs *can* be inserted any day up to day 19 of a 28-day menstrual cycle and they can also be used as a post-coital method (see page 114). However, they are normally fitted during your period. When you first discuss having an IUD, the doctor will need to examine you and may take some swabs to ensure you have no infection. This is because if you do have an infection, having an IUD inserted may increase your risks of pelvic inflammatory disease (PID). PID is when sexual infection passes to the reproductive areas of your body such as the womb, the fallopian tubes and the walls of the pelvic cavity. PID causes inflammation which leads to scarring, and scar tissue can often build up, to bind together your tubes and ovaries. In the worse cases this can lead to infertility.

To have an IUD inserted, you will be asked to remove your lower clothes and to lie on the doctor's couch. You may be asked to lie on your back with your knees pulled up and your feet flat, or curled on your side. The doctor may offer you a painkiller, something to help you relax or a local anaesthetic beforehand. She or he will then give you an internal examination to check that all is well and will pass a speculum into your vagina to do this. A speculum is a plastic or metal device made up of two long, flat and scoop-shaped bowls that are hinged together in a ring. It looks rather like a duck's bill and is designed to hold the walls of your vagina gently apart.

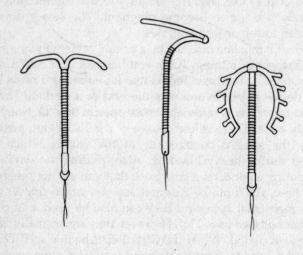

Figures 15a and b: IUDs (intrauterine devices)

The doctor passes the speculum inside your vagina (a few doctors may give it to you to insert yourself). It is then opened out to separate the walls of your vagina and give a good view up to the cervix and to the end of the vagina. The doctor will then use forceps – a blunt, tweezer-like instrument – to hold the cervix steady. You may feel a slight pinch or nip when this is done. A 'sound' – a slim rod – is passed up through the cervix into the womb to measure the womb's length. You may notice a cramping, period-like pain as this is happening.

When you are both ready, the doctor will pass a hollow rod containing the IUD up through the vagina and cervix and into your womb. As the rod is drawn out, it leaves the IUD in place behind. The IUD will have been straightened out in the hollow rod but will open up into its own shape when the rod is removed. The threads will remain hanging down, and these will be trimmed to be just long enough for you to feel with a finger. If they are left too long, you may be aware of them. If

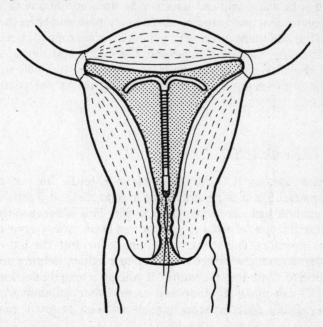

they are left too short, they may be felt by your partner. If this does happen you should go back to the doctor who fitted your IUD for advice.

Having an IUD put in place can take as little as two to three minutes. It might take longer if you feel tense or nervous, and it would be a good idea to give yourself a few minutes to recover afterwards. You may have some cramps or slight bleeding afterwards. Some women feel faint, find their heart races or even slows down unusually. A few minutes' rest are usually all that is needed.

You will be asked to return six to eight weeks later for a check-up, although you should go back sooner if you have any problems or worries. If all is well, you will be given a routine follow-up appointment six months later and then be seen once a year. IUDs can be left in place for some years. Most family planning authorities now recommend that copper IUDs should be left in place for a minimum of five years. Once the device is in place, you can have sex as often and at any time you please. You only need to check every now and then that the IUD is still there. After your period is a good time to check. You do this by passing a finger into the vagina and feeling to see if the threads are still in place. However, you will still benefit from seeing your family planning doctor for yearly checks.

Can I Use an IUD?

You can use an IUD for most of your fertile life up to menopause. But it is generally not a good method if you or your partner have sex with other people. This is because the IUD carries special risks if you are exposed to any type of sexual infection. The strings that hang down into the top of the vagina from the device may act like a ladder, helping any infection to climb into the womb. If you get a sexual infection, the IUD can make it worse and cause Pelvic Inflammatory Disease (PID). Women who have never been pregnant may experience more pain and period problems than those who have been pregnant before having an IUD fitted.

Your doctor needs to know if you have severe heart disease, anaemia or if you are taking drugs that suppress the immune system. An IUD is also unsuitable if you know you are or think you might be pregnant, have an abnormally shaped womb, have already had an ectopic pregnancy, have any infection or had severe PID in the past. Neither would you be recommended to have an IUD if you have heavy, painful periods. If you have no periods at all, the reasons for this would need to be investigated before an IUD could be fitted.

Advantages

The IUD is a 'no fuss', reversible method of female contraception. It starts working as soon as you have it put in and stops as soon as you have it taken out, which makes it ideal for women spacing their pregnancies. It does not interfere with lovemaking.

You make up your mind, you pay one visit to a surgery or clinic and, apart from periodic health checks and ensuring once a month that the device is still in place, you can forget about contraception for several years.

The advantage of the first generation plastic-only IUDs was that they could be left in place until the menopause. Although they are no longer made, any woman who still has one and has no problems can confidently leave it in place until she no longer needs it, with one exception (see the end of the Risks section).

Disadvantages

You have to go to a doctor to get it, and having an IUD put in can be uncomfortable. The IUD may also be expelled or pushed out of the womb. If this happens, you will be at risk of pregnancy at once and should go back to your doctor to have another one fitted. An IUD can produce menstrual changes, such as spotting before and after a period.

Side Effects

Periods may be heavier than usual at first. You may also experience spotting at any time in your cycle. Periods can last longer, starting gradually and then tailing off over a few days, and may also be more painful, with cramps and backaches for some women.

Risks

If you are to have any problems with an IUD, they are likely to happen in the first three to six months of use. Women using IUDs do seem to be more at risk of getting an infection which might lead to PID if they are not in mutually faithful relationships. Some IUD users also have a greater incidence of vaginal discharges. Using an IUD does *not* increase your risks of developing cancer of the cervix or womb.

Rare complications with the IUD are perforation and ectopic pregnancy. Perforation is when the IUD goes through the wall of the womb or the side of the cervix. This is more likely to happen when it is being put in and is often the fault of the inserter. This is why it is so important to have your IUD put in by someone with the proper training and lots of experience. Anyone who does feel any pain or has a difficult fitting and can't feel the threads afterwards, or gets any pain, bleeding or other problems in the abdomen or when passing a motion or water, should go back to their doctor at once.

Ectopic pregnancy is when a fertilized egg does not complete its journey down into the womb, but stops, usually in one of the two fallopian tubes and then embeds and starts developing there. An ectopic pregnancy cannot survive in the fallopian tube as the tube can only stretch so far before it bursts, causing pain and internal bleeding. An immediate operation would be needed to control this. Any light, scanty or missed period with an IUD should *always* be investigated to rule out this possibility.

Many women using one first generation plastic-only IUD – the Dalkon Shield – in the early 1970s were found to suffer infection far more often than normal. Any women who knows she still has a Dalkon Shield in place should have it removed as soon as possible.

Pregnancy and Breastfeeding

If you want to become pregnant, you simply have the device removed. The contraceptive action of the IUD stops immediately it is taken out. There is no effect on a baby if you get pregnant after having an IUD removed.

If you do become pregnant while using an IUD, there is no evidence of any abnormality in babies born as a result. However, you may have an increased possibility of having a miscarriage, so it is advisable to have the IUD removed. The earlier you have the IUD taken out the better, if you do want to continue with the pregnancy. You are advised to see your doctor as soon as you think you are pregnant. If the pregnancy is less than 12 weeks old, if the threads are visible and if the IUD will come out without problems, it will be removed. If the IUD cannot be taken out and the baby goes to full term, the IUD cannot harm it. The device will be lying in between the wall of your womb and the protective sac that surrounds your baby, and will usually be pushed out with the afterbirth.

After childbirth, you would normally need to wait six weeks before having an IUD fitted. Immediately after having a baby there is a higher risk of expulsion. If you are planning to breastfeed, you may be advised or choose to use another method of contraception until your baby is weaned, as breastfeeding may increase your risk of perforation.

CHAPTER SIX

Natural Family Planning

Also known as the rhythm method, the safe period, periodic abstinence, fertility awareness and NFP.

Natural methods rely on the fact that there is actually a very short time in her monthly cycle when a woman can get pregnant. Using one or a mixture of these methods, you try to work out when that time will be and avoid having intercourse: you can make love in ways that do not risk pregnancy or use a barrier method. 'Fertility awareness' means knowing when you are likely to get pregnant and 'periodic abstinence' means going without sexual intercourse at fertile times.

It is likely that human beings have practised periodic abstinence ever since they discovered that sexual intercourse leads to pregnancy. Ancient Greek physicians talked about sterile periods and times when a woman was more likely to get pregnant. However, until the late 1850s, it was thought that the time you had to avoid if you didn't want to get pregnant was just before or during a period. It wasn't until the 1920s to 1930s that ovulation was properly understood.

Around 10 to 15 million couples throughout the world use natural methods. Once an egg has been released, it must meet and join with sperm within 24 hours, at the most, to develop successfully into a baby. This is a woman's fertile period. Sperm can survive for up to seven days in a woman's body, so you would be protected from pregnancy if you make sure you don't make love in the days before and after ovulation. However, it is not always easy to know exactly when you will ovulate each month. Ovulation does not come along at a set number of days *after* a period. But periods do come a fairly regular 12 to 16 days *after* ovulation. So over a time, you may be able to get some idea of when ovulation has happened in previous months, and learn to estimate when it may happen in future months. You can also learn how to notice changes in your body that can tell you when ovulation is about to happen. If a couple want to use fertility awareness in order to avoid pregnancy, they can use this knowledge to know when not to have sex, when to make love in ways that do not risk pregnancy or when to use a barrier method. If a couple are wanting to plan a pregnancy, they can then also use this knowledge to have sex at a time most likely to start a baby.

Results from studies on the effectiveness of natural methods vary a lot. Two out of every hundred couples who are committed to using the method carefully and avoid sex during the fertile times, might have a pregnancy in a year. However, some studies have shown figures nearer to 20 couples in every hundred. The most effective NFP method is using a combination of ways of predicting ovulation, such as the symptothermal method or double-check method. Successful use of natural methods would be increased by the information and help you could receive from a trained NFP teacher. Your own doctor or practice nurse, or a doctor or nurse at a family planning clinic, may be able to help you. However, specialist help is available from the National Family Planning Service or the Natural Family Planning Unit (see Useful Addresses), both of which could supply you with addresses of trained NFP teachers in your area. Once you have learned and become confident with the method, you will not need any follow-up or further teaching. You could, however, go back to your NFP teacher or doctor with any problems or worries and you should continue to see your doctor for routine well woman care.

How Do You Use Natural Methods?

There are four natural family planning methods, that you can use to work out when ovulation is likely to happen each month. Some methods are more effective than others, and some women choose a combination of these methods for greater effectiveness.

Calendar Method

In this method you keep a record of your periods over several months – usually six to 12. The idea is to find out the earliest and the latest you are likely to ovulate, and not have sex at any point that could put you at risk.

To work out your safe and unsafe days, you find out the length of your *shortest* and *longest* cycles in the time you've kept records. You always count the *first* day of a period as day one. Let's say in your shortest month your period started on day 26, and your longest cycle was when your period came on day 35. To calculate the *beginning* of your fertile period, you take 18 from that 26. Then, to calculate the *end* of your fertile period you take 10 from that 35.

Shortest cycle 26 − 18 = 8

Longest cycle 35 − 10 = 25

This would mean that you may get pregnant if you have intercourse at any time from day eight to day 25. If you had intercourse during this time, unless you want to get pregnant, you are advised to use a barrier method of contraception, or use withdrawal or have sex without putting penis in vagina.

The calendar method is not very reliable and is not a recommended method on its own. If you want to use it as a way of protecting you from pregnancy, you should combine it with both of the other methods.

Temperature Method

Hormonal changes in your body during your menstrual cycle

will affect your temperature. This drops very slightly just before your body releases an egg at ovulation. Then, as the level of the hormone progesterone increases, it rises again until a few days before your period, when it drops again as the level of progesterone goes down. If you carefully take and record your temperature, you can see this dip and peak. You can get a special fertility thermometer, which makes this easy to read, prescribed by your doctor or from a chemist. You need to find your Basal Body Temperature (BBT), which means your temperature at rest. You do this by taking your temperature just after you wake up and before you do anything to raise it, such as moving around or having a hot drink. Average body temperature is usually accepted to be 37° Centigrade. You will probably find that your temperature normally ranges between 36.5°C and 37.2°C and your BBT is usually lower. The important change to notice is a rise of some 0.2°C to 0.4°C, which will happen just after ovulation.

After three days in a row where your temperature was higher than the previous six days, you are safe to have sex. The egg will have been released and will no longer be able to be fertilized from this point on. If you take your temperature regularly and keep a chart and your cycles are steady, you may feel confident enough to predict when ovulation is going to occur. You can then have sex in the early part of your cycle and only stop when the fertile time comes.

Cervical Mucus Or Billings Method

The amount and type of moisture you have in your vagina and especially around the neck of the womb changes during your monthly cycle. Just after your period you are likely to have several days when you may feel dry. The cervical mucus will be thick and sticky and form a plug around the cervix. This serves as a barrier to sperm. After a few days, as ovulation approaches, the cervix begins to produce more mucus and the amount increases up until a peak day. This fertile mucus is

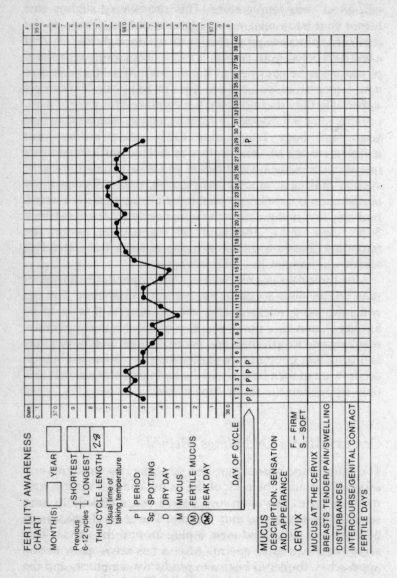

Figure 16: An example of a temperature chart

thinner and more slippery. Instead of blocking the passage of sperm, its job is to make a pregnancy more likely. So it forms channels to encourage sperm to swim through the cervical canal into the womb. Fertile mucus is nourishing to sperm, allowing it to live longer and swim faster. After the peak day, the cervical mucus quickly returns to being sticky and dry, again forming a barrier to sperm at the cervix.

You can learn to recognize these changes and the signs that ovulation is about to happen and so avoid the fertile time. You may notice these by how you feel, or by how much mucus you find on your underpants or when you wipe yourself dry after a visit to the loo, but the best way is by a finger test. As ovulation approaches and mucus starts to increase, you would find it to be a creamy, sticky consistency. It may be quite thick and a cloudy white or yellow colour. If you rub some between finger and thumb, and then stretch them apart, the mucus will break up.

As you get nearer to ovulation, the mucus increases in amount and becomes thinner, more watery and more stretchy. At your most fertile time the cervical mucus will be slippery and elastic and have the appearance and feel of raw egg white. It may stretch several inches on the finger and thumb test before breaking. After ovulation, mucus becomes sticky, cloudy or white and then scant again. Since the dry days are your infertile time, you are able to have sex during them, but will be risking pregnancy if you have intercourse during the fertile time.

Symptothermal or Double-Check Method

The best option for using natural methods effectively is to combine them. To use this symptothermal or double-check method you can take your temperature and look at your cervical mucus each day, and keep careful records of the results. You could also learn to notice other symptoms that can tell you about changes in your body during your monthly cycle. Many women get pain when they ovulate. This is called Mittelschmerz (German for 'middle pain') and can be a gripping ache, usually on one side of the lower abdomen. You may also have a few spots of blood from the vagina at the same time. Noticing any blood, breast tenderness or mood changes can all be ways you can tune in to your own cycle.

There are now ovulation testing kits, available in the UK from pharmacies, which are aimed at people wanting to plan a pregnancy. These are urine tests that allow you to detect the sudden surge in luteinizing hormone, the hormone that increases about 24 hours before ovulation. They would, however, be an expensive way to predict ovulation each month in order to avoid a pregnancy.

Can I Use Natural Methods?

Provided you are happy to make all the necessary checks and keep accurate and detailed records, anyone can use natural methods. You can use natural methods from the time your periods became regular up to the menopause. At certain points in a woman's life more care will be needed in understanding the signals her body is giving her, for instance after the birth of a baby or as she approaches menopause.

Advantages

There are no changes imposed on the body, pills or mechanical devices involved. The methods are easy to learn, and once learned nothing else is needed. Natural methods are always at hand and don't affect the sex act itself. Knowing about the woman's cycle can help you understand more about your own body. It can also help you plan your family when you *do* want to get pregnant.

The best advantage of natural family planning is that it can actually help bring a couple together and make sex very special and exciting. You may find yourself eagerly waiting and planning for your infertile days and discovering other ways of pleasing each other than penis-in-vagina sex on your fertile days. Talking together about your sexual needs and pregnancy can also help you to share and discuss many other aspects of your life together.

Disadvantages

Natural methods do need commitment, co-operation and planning for them to work for you. You need to see a specially trained teacher, who may be a nurse or doctor, in order to best learn how to use the methods.

Side Effects
There are no side effects from using NFP methods.

Risks
None.

Pregnancy and Breastfeeding

One advantage of natural methods is that when you do want to become pregnant, you can use the knowledge you have about your fertile days to plan when you *will* make love. Your having used natural methods will have no effect on a baby when you do fall pregnant.

Natural methods have no effect on breastfeeding. They can also be particularly useful in pinpointing when you become fertile again. Full breastfeeding (two to four-hourly, day and night) may prevent ovulation for as long as you continue to feed in this way.

Withdrawal

Also known as pulling out, being careful, coitus interruptus.

Withdrawal or 'pulling out' is when the man pulls his penis out of his partner's vagina just before he comes. If the man comes outside the woman, sperm has less chance of travelling through the womb into the fallopian tubes and meeting up with a waiting egg. It is a very ancient method, mentioned in the Bible in the story of Onan who 'spilled his seed on the ground' to avoid a pregnancy.

In some countries where other methods are hard to obtain, withdrawal is the main method of birth control. It is particularly well-used in Catholic countries and in Eastern Europe. Around four per cent of couples use it regularly in the UK, but it is almost certainly more popular than statistics suggest. Many young people use it before seeking advice on contraception, and many people of all ages fall back on it if they forget pills, lose their diaphragm or cap or run out of condoms.

Withdrawal is not always a very effective method, especially if it is being used by default rather than from positive choice. Between eight and 25 women will get pregnant out of 100 couples using this method over a year. One problem with withdrawal is that viable sperm can be found in the lubrication produced by the man even before he comes.

How Do You Use Withdrawal?

The couple have sex until the man feels he is about to come. He then pulls his penis out of her vagina and comes outside her.

Can I Use Withdrawal?

You can use withdrawal at any time in your fertile life, but you may find it difficult in the early days. Knowing when to pull out and having the self-control to do so can be hard.

Withdrawal is an unreliable proposition for young and inexperienced lovers, or for couples in the first flush of love. The less experienced or more excited you are, the more likely you are to misjudge things and come while still inside.

Advantages

Withdrawal doesn't cost anything, is drug-free, is always on hand and needs no preparation or equipment. You can use it at any time of the month.

Disadvantages

Unless it is a positive choice, using withdrawal can lead to stress, tension and unhappiness. You have to use a large amount of self-control at the very moments when you might want to lose it totally. Withdrawal has a high failure rate.

Side Effects
Knowing that he will have to withdraw can affect both partners' pleasure.

Risks
None.

Pregnancy and Breastfeeding

If you want to get pregnant, simply stop using the method. Having used withdrawal should have no effect on a baby, and you can use withdrawal during breastfeeding.

CHAPTER SEVEN

Surgical Methods

Sterilization is an operation which permanently leaves a woman unable to become pregnant or a man unable to cause a pregnancy. It has *no* other effect, and both men and women are still able to enjoy sex and a woman will continue to have periods. The first recorded female sterilization was done in 1881, and the first recorded male sterilization or vasectomy in 1894.

Worldwide, over 100 million people have been sterilized, and one in three couples who use some form of contraception rely on female sterilization or vasectomy. In the UK, three million people are sterilized, of which half are men and half women. In the USA, the figure is 9.5 million with the same almost equal split between the sexes. In India, men are more likely to opt for this operation and the proportion there is two-thirds men to one-third women, but in Canada only two per cent of the million sterilized people are male.

Female Sterilization

Also known as tubal ligation or having your tubes tied.

Female sterilization is almost completely effective. The failure rate is 0.1–0.3 per cent; that is, between one and three women in 1,000 may get pregnant after being sterilized, depending on the method used. The more experienced the surgeon, the less the chance of failure.

In female sterilization, the fallopian tubes – the tubes that carry the egg from the ovaries to the womb – are blocked, sealed or cut. Eggs continue to be released each month but are absorbed by the body quite normally and harmlessly. You may go in for a 'day care' operation or to stay overnight. Most of these operations are done under a light general anaesthetic, where you are put to sleep. Sometimes a local anaesthetic may be offered. Some operations need only one or two tiny cuts in the abdomen, usually one in the navel and one slightly lower down, just below the top of your pubic hair. The hair will be shaved off only in the area around the cut. Most sterilizing operations done on women in the Western world are now performed using an instrument called a laparoscope. This acts like a telescope, and looks very much like one. It is a metal instrument that uses fibre optics to shine a light into the body while sending back a clear picture from a tiny camera to the surgeon operating. Some surgeons use a type of laparoscope that allows them to pass their operating instruments down the laparoscope itself, so only needing one cut to be made. Others pass the laparoscope through one cut and the operating instruments through another. In a few cases the operation may be done through an inside cut in the top of the vagina. Vaginal operations do not leave a visible scar, but carry a higher risk of post-operative infection. This route is usually only used for good medical reasons, such as when the patient is very overweight or the abdomen is already heavily scarred. Sometimes, the surgeon will need to make a bigger incision for a clearer view. If so a mini-laparotomy is performed, with one horizontal cut just below the bikini line used.

Whichever technique is used, the surgeon will locate the fallopian tubes and then cut them and either remove a section or seal the cut ends to close them up. An alternative technique is to put clips or tiny rubber bands on the fallopian tubes to close them tightly shut. Sometimes the cut is so small it only needs to be taped shut. The operation is effective immediately. Once you have recovered from it, you can have sex as often and whenever you choose.

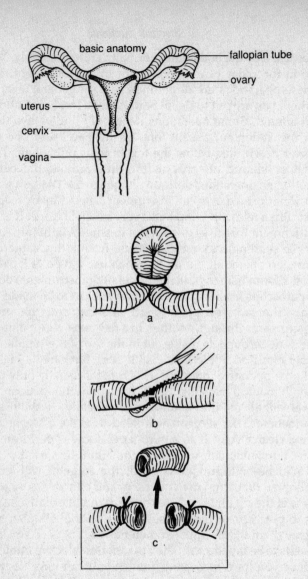

Figure 17: Female sterilization. The fallopian tubes are blocked
with a ring (a), or a clip (b), or cut (c).

Can I Have the Operation?

Your doctor will need to know whether you have any problems in the female reproductive organs that would make the operation difficult. When you see your doctor to discuss sterilization, an examination may therefore be done. An opportunity to discuss your decision should also be offered, since sterilization may be regretted if you have any sexual or emotional problems in the relationship or are not certain about your decision. You are unlikely to be offered a sterilization if you are younger than 25. Women who have any medical reasons for being advised not to have a general anaesthetic, or are overweight, may find this affects the type of operation offered. You are also advised not to have a female sterilization at the same time as having a baby or an abortion. Neither are good times to make such an irrevocable decision. You or your doctor may think it a good idea to combine two hospital stays into one, but you have a greater than normal risk of sterilization failure if you have the operation done after a birth. This is because the blood supply to the fallopian tubes is very rich at this time and this can encourage the tubes to heal up and rejoin by themselves.

You may choose to ask for sterilization if you have medical reasons for not wanting to become pregnant, such as an inherited disease or ill health. Most people opting for sterilization have children. You may choose to be sterilized at an earlier age when you have had only one child or no children at all. Sterilization should be considered to be irreversible and once you have had the operation it *is* your method of contraception for life. For that reason you may like to take some time thinking about and discussing the reasons for your choice and the other options. You may find it particularly helpful to talk these through with a professional, such as a doctor, nurse or counsellor. You will need to consider whether your feelings may change if your present relationship ends or, if you have children, if one or more of them were to die. Sterilization is only suitable if you are sure you will not want to become pregnant afterwards. If the *possibility* that sex might result in pregnancy is important to you, sterilization would not be a good idea.

Advantages

Sterilization is the most effective birth control method of all. Once you have made up your mind and had the operation, you need never worry about contraception again. There are no health risks to having been sterilized. Women do not put on weight or lose their femininity or sexual urges. You may find you are happier and healthier as a result of no longer having to worry about unwanted pregnancy. Sterilization also has the special advantage of being the one method that *either* partner can choose.

Disadvantages

It *is* permanent in many cases and you can never guarantee you might be able to reverse your decision. The operation can be painful or uncomfortable, and afterwards a few women may have heavier or altered periods. The cut tubes can rejoin by themselves, or a surgeon might even cut something else by mistake, leaving you fertile. Then, you can be at risk of pregnancy. This is, however, very rare.

Side Effects
Studies show that one side effect of sterilization is more sex. Newly sterilized couples make love more often after their operation than before. Whether this is because they no longer need to worry about pregnancy or because they feel they have to prove the operation has had no effect on their urges, we don't know.

Some women complain of heavier, painful periods after sterilization. This may be because they had been using the Pill for some time and had got used to the lighter and pain-free bleeds this can produce. Periods can alter and become heavier and more painful as you get older, so it might be the passage of time that makes them worse rather than the sterilization operation itself. However, it has been suggested that interfering with blood flow in the pelvis by cutting and sealing the fallopian tubes may itself alter period patterns. This seems not to be such a problem with methods that involve blocking the fallopian tubes, such as rings or clips.

Risks
There are always risks in having a general anaesthetic. During the female operation other parts of her body next to the fallopian tubes, such as the bowel, can be damaged by mistake. With some methods, the opening cut and the internal surgery can also be painful. In the rare occasions when a pregnancy does occur after sterilization, there is a higher risk of its being ectopic.

There is no evidence to show that women who have sterilizations are any more likely to suffer any ill health because of the operation. Certainly the health risks to a woman of an unplanned pregnancy outweigh the health risks of sterilization.

Changing Your Mind

It is important not to opt for sterilization if you have *any* doubts, or thoughts of wanting to get pregnant again. If you did want to do so, reversal operations are not always available on the NHS and you would have to pay for a costly private operation or convince a doctor that a reversal operation was justified.

There is no guarantee that this second operation would be successful.

Having said that, some sterilizations can and have been reversed. Some sterilization methods have a slightly higher rate of success when reversed. These are the ones that cause as little damage as possible to the fallopian tubes. If, instead of cutting and sealing tubes, clips were used, a skilful surgeon could trim ends and rejoin the cut tubes at a later date. However, pregnancies to mothers who have had a reversal operation are more likely to be ectopic because scar tissue in the fallopian tubes may result in a fertilized egg being unable to complete its journey to the womb. But there is no evidence that babies born to women after a sterilization failure or a successful reversal are any more likely to have problems than before the operation.

New developments in microsurgery have increased the success rate of attempted reversals to between 30 and 70 per cent. If clips were used, the success rate can be as high as 80 per cent. The length of time between having had your sterilization and an attempted reversal may make a difference, in that if the sterilization was done some years ago it is more likely to have involved cutting and removing more of the tube than would be done today. Also, the older you are the less fertile you will be.

Breastfeeding

Although it isn't a good idea to make decisions about, or have a sterilization at the same time as giving birth, if you do so you can be reassured the operation will have no effect on breastfeeding.

Male Sterilization

Also known as vasectomy, the cut or the snip.

Vasectomy is even more effective than female sterilizations, with about 0.1 per cent of operations failing – one in 1,000. As with female sterilizations, the more experienced the surgeon, the less the chance of failure.

In vasectomy, the vas deferens – the tubes that carry the sperm from the testes to the penis – are cut or sealed. Sperm are still produced but are absorbed by the body quite normally and harmlessly, as they would be if the man did not ejaculate through having sex, masturbating or having wet dreams. With a few exceptions, vasectomies are done under local anaesthetic as 'day-care' cases. This means that you go to the surgery, clinic or hospital and can expect to walk out in as little as half an hour with the operation completed.

To have the operation, you would be asked to shave around your genitals. You would be given a small injection of anaesthetic in one side of your scrotum. The surgeon would make a tiny cut in the scrotum, find the vas and cut it. A piece of the vas may be removed, or the ends sealed and tied back on themselves. The cut ends are then buried back in the tissues of the scrotum and the cut closed with one or several stitches. Since this cut is so small, stitches are not always needed and sometimes it only needs to be sealed with surgical tape. The whole procedure is then repeated for the other side of the scrotum. Some surgeons use the same incision for both sides. In a new technique, the surgeon can use specially designed forceps to make a tiny puncture. The loose skin of the scrotum is then stretched and both vas reached through this one hole. This 'no scalpel' technique does not need stitches and reportedly produces less pain or bruising than conventional surgery.

After a rest, you can go home. You would need to have several sperm counts to make sure that no sperm still remain in the tubes. Specimens can either be taken or sent to a laboratory for this. It can take many ejaculations – about 24 to 36 – for the sperm to clear from the tubes. So although you can have sex as soon as you feel comfortable, the couple must use other methods of contraception until the man has given two sperm samples that show that no sperm are getting through. You can't tell just by looking at your own ejaculate whether sperm are present or not. You still produce the same amount of semen, and it is unchanged in appearance. After

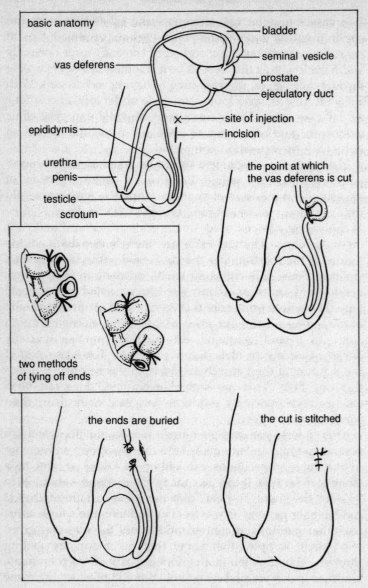

Figure 18: Vasectomy (male sterilization)

the 'all clear' is given, you can make love as often and whenever you choose without needing additional contraception.

Can I Have the Operation?

Your doctor would need to know whether you had any problems in the male reproductive organs that would make the operation difficult and may offer an examination to make sure all is well. You are unlikely to be offered a vasectomy if you are younger than 25. You may also be advised not to have a vasectomy at the same time as your partner is having a baby or an abortion. Neither are good times to make such an irrevocable decision.

You may choose to ask for vasectomy if you have medical reasons for not wanting to cause a pregnancy, such as an inherited disease or ill health. Most people opting for vasectomy have children. You may choose to be sterilized at an earlier age when you have had only one child or no children at all. Vasectomy should be considered to be irreversible and once you have had the operation it *is* your method of contraception for life. For that reason, you may like to take some time thinking about and discussing the reasons for your choice and the other options. You may find it particularly helpful to talk these through with a professional, such as a doctor, nurse or counsellor. You will need to consider whether your feelings may change if your present relationship ends or, if you have children, if one or more of them were to die. It is also not advisable to consider vasectomy if your relationship is in crisis or you have any sexual problems. Vasectomy is only suitable if you are sure you will not want to father a child afterwards. If the *possibility* that sex might result in pregnancy is important to you, vasectomy would not be a good idea.

Advantages

Vasectomy is the most effective birth control method of all.
Once you have made up your mind and had the operation,
you need never worry about contraception again. There are no
health risks to having been sterilized and, in spite of the 'scare'
stories', men do not get cancer, age more quickly, become
unable to make love or lose any sexual urges. You may be
happier and healthier as a result of no longer having to worry
about unwanted pregnancy. Sterilization also has the special
advantage of being the one method that *either* partner can
choose.

Disadvantages

Vasectomy *is* permanent in many cases and you can never
guarantee you might be able to reverse your decision. The
operation can be painful or uncomfortable. You will need a few
days off work immediately afterwards and there may be
swelling, bruising and discomfort. You will need to wear
supportive underwear and rest with your feet up for a day or
so. Vasectomy isn't foolproof immediately and you need to
have had two clear sperm tests before you can rely on it. The
cut tubes can rejoin by themselves, or a surgeon might even
cut something else by mistake, leaving you still fertile. Then
your partner can be at risk of pregnancy. This is, however, very
rare.

Side Effects
Studies show that one side effect of sterilization is more sex.
Newly sterilized couples make love more often after their
operation than before. Whether this is because they no longer
need to worry about pregnancy, or because they feel they have
to prove the operation has had no effect on their urges, we
don't know.

After a vasectomy, the immune system might react to sperm

as if it were a foreign, harmful substance and start killing them by producing antibodies. You will not notice any difference unless you decide to try for a reversal operation. The operation may succeed, but these changes may make it more difficult for you to make a woman pregnant. Sexual ability and enjoyment, however, is unchanged.

Risks
There are always risks in having a general anaesthetic. This is why it is better for a vasectomy to be carried out under local anaesthesia. And why, if all things *are* equal, it might be better for the man in a couple to be sterilized rather than his partner – if the choice is between a vasectomy under a local anaesthetic or a female sterilization under general. A tiny lump, a sperm granuloma, often develops at the end of the vas. Sometimes, nerves can get trapped in this and the area can ache and be tender and painful. In many cases, no treatment is necessary but sometimes the sperm granuloma may need to be removed with a minor operation.

There is no evidence to show that men who have vasectomies are any more likely to suffer any ill health because of the operations. There have been some reports that men who have vasectomies have a higher risk of developing prostate and testicular cancer, but the conclusion from all the research published at present shows that these cancers were probably caused by factors other than the vasectomy itself. There have also been suggestions that vasectomy may increase your risk of having kidney stones, although this has not been confirmed by other studies.

Changing Your Mind

It is important not to opt for vasectomy if you have *any* doubts, or thoughts of wanting to make your partner pregnant again. If you did want to change your mind, reversal operations are not always available on the NHS and you would have to pay

for a costly private operation or convince a doctor that a
reversal operation was justified. There are the usual risks
associated with any operation and there is no guarantee that
this second operation would be successful.

Having said that, vasectomies can and have been reversed.
Some sterilization methods have a slightly higher rate of
success when reversed. These are the ones that cause as little
damage as possible to the vas. If the vas were cut and tied
without being sealed or any length removed, a skilful surgeon
could trim ends and rejoin the cut tubes at a later date.

New developments in microsurgery have increased the
success rate of attempted reversals. However, the length of
time in between the two operations can be vitally important.
The body can start producing antibodies to sperm after a few
years. This has no ill effects on your health or sexual ability,
but it may mean that even if a reversal is successful in physical
terms – and more than 90 per cent of attempts at reconnecting
the vas are – these sperm may not be able to fertilize an egg.
The pregnancy rate after reversal is around 30 per cent. After
10 years the chances of success are less.

CHAPTER EIGHT

Emergency Contraception

Also known as post-coital contraception.

Emergency or post-coital (after-sex) contraception is a way of stopping a pregnancy after you've had unprotected sex. It is a method of contraception which works before a pregnancy starts, rather than a type of abortion, which happens after a pregnancy has begun.

We all make mistakes. Sometimes a method of birth control fails: a condom breaks or an IUD comes out. Or we get caught up in passion and leave the diaphragm in the bathroom cabinet or the condom in a pocket. You may have forgotten to pack your pills before going on holiday or find the dog (or the baby) has chewed your cap to pieces, and think 'We'll risk it, just this once.'

After-sex methods have been tried for centuries. Jumping up and down or sneezing after sex have long been suggested as ways of avoiding pregnancy. So have washing out the vagina with mixtures of salt water, vinegar or wine, or crouching over incense to allow the smoke to enter the vagina. Unfortunately, since sperm can be found in the womb 90 seconds after ejaculation, and in the fallopian tubes within five minutes, you would have to move very sharply to catch them. In fact, squirting water or any liquid into the vagina after sex is more likely to force sperm *up* into the womb and can also lead to infections. Since the 1960s, more effective methods have been found.

Emergency contraception does not try to stop the meeting of sperm and egg, which can happen as little as five minutes after climax. Instead, it is a way of preventing a fertilized egg from reaching the womb at the right time for it to implant itself there and begin to develop, and of preventing it from embedding in the lining of the womb. There are two ways to do this. One is to take a special dose of combined contraceptive pills. The other is to have an IUD inserted. Both methods will only work effectively and safely if done within a certain time limit. The post-coital pill must be taken not later than three days (72 hours) after having unprotected sex. You have more leeway with the IUD. This should be put in within five days (120 hours) of unprotected sex, although it will also be effective if inserted not later than five days after ovulation.

If taken early enough in the menstrual cycle, the post-coital pill can work by delaying ovulation so that by the time you do ovulate, sperm would no longer be able to fertilize an egg. If ovulation is not delayed, taking the post-coital pill has the same effects as having an IUD put in at the right time. That is, they change the speed at which the egg is wafted down the fallopian tube into the womb. A fertilized egg needs to take seven days on its journey down into the womb to develop to the right stage to be able to embed in the lining. If it gets there too early, the egg will not be ready and will pass out of the womb to be washed away in body fluids. Pills and IUD will also affect the lining of the womb, making it unwelcoming to a fertilized egg. Having had an IUD put in, your period should come on time. After taking the emergency pills, your period might be early, on time or a few days late. Ovulation may not happen for at least six weeks after taking the pills.

Emergency contraception is a very good way of preventing pregnancy after the fact. But it is not foolproof, and the Pill taken in this way is less effective than using most other methods in a regular way. Up to four in every 100 women using the Pill correctly as emergency contraception may become pregnant, and less than one in every 100 will become pregnant after having an emergency IUD inserted.

How Do You Use Emergency Contraception?

Whether you are going to be prescribed the post-coital pill or an IUD, you will need to see a doctor and have a full discussion. When you ask to see a doctor for emergency contraception it is very important to say that this is the reason for your visit. This ensures you can be given an immediate appointment. You will need to go through the same health checks and discussion that you would if you were being put on the combined pill or given the IUD for regular birth control. Conditions or problems that may stop you using either the Pill or the IUD as your usual method of contraception would not necessarily make them unsuitable for you as an emergency method. But if one of them is unsuitable, the other may be acceptable. The doctor, to be able to help you, will need to know the date of your last period, exactly when you had unprotected sex and whether you have had unprotected sex at any other time since your last period. This information helps the doctor work out whether you were at risk of pregnancy or whether you might already be pregnant from a previous act of unprotected sex, so the appropriate treatment can be given. You would be asked to return for a follow-up visit around the time when your next period is expected.

Post-Coital Pill

You will see a doctor who will give or prescribe for you a dose of four pills. You take two of these *at once*, not later than three days (72 hours) after having unprotected sex. You take the other two pills 12 hours after the first dose – no more, no less. This timing is so important that you may need to set an alarm clock to wake you up, if the second dose is to be taken when you are asleep. If you are within the 72 hour limit when you see your doctor, and taking the pills at that time would mean you have to take the second dose when you would otherwise be asleep, you may start the treatment a few hours later.

This is *not* a do-it-yourself method. You can't make it work with your own or a friend's combined pill. The combined pill that most people have is the wrong dose and it simply won't have the right effect.

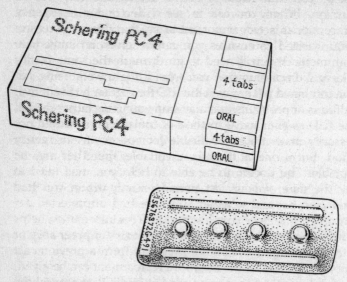

Figure 19: The post-coital pill

The IUD

You would visit a doctor and have an IUD inserted. This may be done up to five days (120 hours) after having unprotected sex. If you are any later than that, but by your and your doctor's calculation are still within five days after ovulation, an IUD may still be inserted.

Can I Use Emergency Methods?

If there are medical reasons for you not being able to use the Pill or the IUD as methods of contraception, you may not be able to use them as an emergency method either.

You will not be able to use emergency contraception if you are too late. But don't forget that although you must be within 72 hours for pills to be started, you do have a longer period within which an IUD can be inserted.

Emergency contraception is not effective enough to be something you rely on every month. It is a one-off method of dealing with an accident or a mistake. Of course, if you have an IUD inserted you can keep it in and settle on that as your future method. But if the reason you needed emergency contraception was because you weren't using any other method, you could make your visit to the doctor a chance to talk over a regular method. And if seeking emergency contraception was because you were making mistakes with your present method, you could talk that over too. Some doctors only feel it is right to give emergency contraception if you were raped or have had an accident with a regular method. However, most doctors would far rather you asked for emergency contraception than waited and then asked for an abortion.

Advantages

If you have been put at risk of an unplanned pregnancy, emergency contraception can avoid the possible need for an abortion later on.

Disadvantages

You have to see a doctor within the very strict time limits – 72 hours for pills and 120 hours for the IUD. It is *not* a method to rely on for more than occasional emergency use. Post-coital pills are less effective than using other methods on a regular basis.

Side Effects

Using the pills, you may feel nauseous and may be sick. This is more likely to happen after the second dose. It's best not to take the pills on an empty stomach, so swallow them after food. Even a few dry biscuits will help. If you are actually sick within three hours of taking a dose, you may need to go back to your doctor at once for another, since the pills may not have been absorbed. You may be given anti-sickness pills and a spare dose of post-coital pills in case this happens. With the IUD, the effects are the same as for a routine IUD insertion (see page 88).

Risks

Since the post-coital pill is a very short course of tablets, the risk from this method is very small. The risks for using an IUD are the same as for having an IUD inserted as a regular contraceptive method.

Pregnancy and Breastfeeding

If the post-coital pill fails and you became pregnant, research to date suggests there are no effects on a baby. Research looking at women who took ordinary oral contraceptive pills during early pregnancy shows no harmful effects. Pregnancies that continue after an emergency IUD has been put in are at the same risk as those to ordinary IUD users (see page 88).

Since a very small amount of the pill hormones gets into mother's milk, and an emergency dose is only over a 12-hour period, there is no reason why you can't go on breastfeeding if you have already established this. If you were worried, you could express some milk before taking the pills and bottle feed for that day. The oestrogen in the pills may, however, affect your milk flow and the amount you produce, which is why you will not be able to use the post-coital pill if you have only just started breastfeeding.

CHAPTER NINE

Unplanned Pregnancy

If contraception fails, or you haven't used a method and emergency contraception has not filled the gap, you may be faced with an unplanned pregnancy. There are three choices that are open to you. You could have the baby and keep it. You could have the baby and offer it for adoption. Or you could have an abortion.

This is not an easy decision to make, and you may find it extremely helpful to ask for counselling. This is where you speak to a professional – a doctor, a nurse or a specialist counsellor – who will help you look at the options and work out which one would be best for you. Counsellors do not tell you what to do or put any pressure on you, but allow you to discuss your situation and your feelings and come to your own conclusion. You may find this sort of help at your own family doctor's surgery, a family planning clinic, one of the pregnancy counselling charities or a youth advisory centre. You may also find counselling help at Relate or from a counsellor or counselling agency suggested by the British Association For Counselling. (See Useful Addresses.)

Your first move, however, would be to find out if you *are* pregnant. You could have a pregnancy test done at various places, each offering advantages and disadvantages.

You could go to any of the following.

Your Own Family Doctor's Surgery
If your doctor offers pregnancy tests – and many GPs do not – the advantages are that the test would be free and you would be assured of confidentiality. Whatever the result of the test, you could be given advice, help and support. The

disadvantages are that only some GPs offer on-the-spot testing and if yours does not, it can take as long as a week for the result to come back to you. Also, some GPs may not be willing to refer you for abortion if their personal beliefs are against it.

A Family Planning Clinic

The advantages are the same as with a family doctor. That is, that the test would be free and you would be assured of confidentiality. Advice, help and support could be offered whatever the result. Most clinics offering this service give an on-the-spot-result. The disadvantage is that many clinics only offer tests to women who are already receiving advice or contraception from them. Many family planning clinics cannot offer direct referral for abortion and would refer you back to your GP.

A Youth Advisory Centre

The advantages are that the test is usually free and you are assured of confidentiality. Help, advice and support will be offered and you would get an on-the-spot result. The disadvantage is that there may not be such a centre near you, and if there is it may not be able to refer you directly for an abortion.

A Pregnancy Counselling Charity

The advantages are that you are assured of confidentiality. Help, advice and support are given and you will receive an on-the-spot result. The disadvantage is that you usually have to pay for the test and for counselling.

A Private Testing Service

The advantages are that the service is confidential and quick. The disadvantages are that you will have to pay for the test and will receive no help or support.

A Pharmacist

The advantages are that there is likely to be a pharmacy near you offering this service and that it will be a quick result. The disadvantage would be that you have to pay for the test. Although pharmacists will offer information and advice, they will not be able to give support or refer for abortion.

Home Pregnancy Testing Kits
The advantages are that the result will be very quick and may be done at an earlier stage than that offered by some of the other services. The disadvantages are that these tests can be expensive and there will be no help or support. You have to follow instructions carefully to avoid getting a wrong result.

Life and Other Anti-Abortion Charities
The advantages are that the test will be free and you will get a quick result. They also offer support during pregnancy and afterwards. The disadvantage is that these charities disapprove of abortion.

Home testing pregnancy kits will be able to tell you whether or not you are pregnant from the day your period is late. Some of the places listed above will offer tests that can give you a result at that stage, but with others you may have to wait up to two weeks after your period is late before having your test. Since, whatever your decision, it is important that you take action as soon as possible, you should not delay before finding out about and getting a pregnancy test.

Having Your Baby and Keeping It

If you decide to have your baby and keep it, it is very important that you see your family doctor (GP) as soon as possible, for advice, help and support through your pregnancy and to receive good antenatal care. Your doctor will also be able to put you in touch with any extra help you may need if, for instance, you do not have the support and encouragement of a partner or your family. You could get help from a health visitor, social services and various voluntary organizations such as the National Council for One Parent Families (see Useful Addresses).

Having Your Baby and Offering It for Adoption

If you decide to have your baby but feel unable to keep it, you should still see your family doctor as soon as possible for advice, help and support through your pregnancy. Your doctor will be able to contact the adoption and fostering section of your local social services, or a local voluntary adoption agency, or put you in touch with the British Agencies for Adoption and Fostering. They can put you in touch with adoption agencies in your area. You can, of course, go directly to any of these agencies.

Having an Abortion

Also known as termination of pregnancy or TOP.

Abortion is a medical procedure to end a pregnancy *after* a fertilized egg has implanted in the lining of the womb. Abortion must be carried out *before* the fetus develops past a certain point. This is generally agreed to be when the fetus could survive outside the mother's womb. In the UK this was understood to be after 28 weeks, but new advances in the care of premature babies have meant that 24 weeks is now the allowed date, except when the mother's health would be at risk or the baby would be badly handicapped. Pregnancies are calculated from day one of your *last* period. However, it is very unusual for a pregnancy to be terminated as late as 24 weeks. Because it can be difficult to work out the date of the last period before a pregnancy began – mistakes are often made here – most doctors in the UK are now reluctant to operate after 20 weeks, and most NHS hospitals will not act after 12 weeks.

An abortion is allowed in Britain if two doctors agree that continuing the pregnancy would risk the physical or emotional health of the mother or existing children, or if the baby would otherwise be born with problems. In some other countries abortion is allowed up to 12 weeks after the last period to any women who asks for the operation.

Around 190,000 abortions a year are carried out on women living in the UK. In countries where contraception *is* difficult to get, abortion may be used as the only way of controlling fertility, even if it is illegal and dangerous. There is no evidence to suggest that women or men take abortion lightly or use it by choice as a method of birth control in countries where contraception and abortion are legal and available.

How Does Abortion Work?
There are two basic methods of abortion: surgical methods and medical methods.

Surgical Methods

There are several ways an abortion can be performed by surgery. In pregnancies of up to 12 weeks, vacuum aspiration or dilatation and curettage (D and C) will be used.

In vacuum aspiration, a narrow, hollow tube is passed through the cervix into the womb. The tube is then attached to a pump and the womb is emptied by gentle pressure. A light general anaesthetic is usually used although in some cases the procedure is done with a local anaesthetic. There have been a few reported cases of women having vacuum aspiration abortions and later finding the pregnancy has continued. This is very rare, but the follow-up appointment with a doctor after the operation would rule this out, as well as checking that all is well with you.

In dilatation and curettage, the cervix is dilated (gently stretched open), and the womb is emptied using a spoon-shaped instrument called a curette. This is usually done under a general anaesthetic.

In most hospitals or clinics, you would stay overnight after, and sometimes also before, an abortion. In some hospitals or clinics, abortions in the first 12 weeks of pregnancy – also known as the first trimester – may be done as day-care operations. This means that as long as there have been no problems, you are allowed to go home a few hours after the operation. If you live more than two hours away from the hospital or clinic, have no-one to stay with you, or you or the doctor feel it would be ill-advised for you to go home, you would stay overnight.

There are two surgical methods of abortion that can be used in a pregnancy that is over 12 weeks. From 12 to about 16 weeks, a dilatation and evacuation (D and E) may be performed. Since the pregnancy is more advanced, the cervix will need to be dilated further and the contents of the womb removed by surgical instruments. The second method is to use chemicals called prostaglandins which bring on a miscarriage. The prostaglandins are given in an injection or by an intravenous drip. When a drip is used, a needle is placed in a vein and then connected to a bottle or plastic bag of prostaglandin solution and the contents are allowed to pass slowly into your body. The chemical can also be delivered by putting a pessary – a solid, tampon-shaped piece of gel – in the vagina. Some hours after the chemical has entered the body, labour will begin. A D and C may also be performed after labour is completed, to make sure all the contents of the womb have been passed.

You would usually stay for two nights in the hospital or clinic when having an abortion done after 12 weeks – also known as the second trimester – of pregnancy.

After an abortion done by any of the surgical methods, you would be asked to come back for a follow-up visit some weeks later, at a time agreed between you and your doctor, to check that all is well.

Medical Methods

A new method of abortion uses anti-progestogens such as mifepristone. This method, which can be used for early abortions of up to nine weeks, involves three stages after initial discussion, counselling and health checks. Whether you smoke, your age and your state of health will all be important factors. The first stage is a prescribed dose of mifepristone, taken under the supervision of a hospital doctor or a doctor in a clinic licensed to carry out abortions. Mifepristone works by softening the cervix and blocking the production of progesterone which is needed to maintain a pregnancy. You would be asked to stay in the hospital or clinic for two hours, to make sure you did not lose the tablets by being sick. You would then go home and may have vaginal bleeding at some time over the next 48 hours.

Two days after taking the tablets, you would return to the hospital or clinic. In a few people, the single dose of tablets will have terminated the pregnancy. Most women, however, go on to the second stage of treatment which involves having a prostaglandin pessary inserted into the vagina. You would stay in the hospital or clinic for four to six hours after having the pessary, but need not necessarily be in a hospital bed. The prostaglandin pessary increases contractions and during this time you would probably experience heavy bleeding. In most cases, the abortion is completed before you leave. The treatment is effective in 95 per cent of cases, and the few women who do not respond to it would have a D and C at this stage.

You would return seven days later for the third and final stage, which is an examination to make sure that all is well.

Side Effects
After an abortion you may bleed and have cramps for a few days. Infection is a risk, so you won't be able to have sex, use tampons, lie in a bath or go swimming until after bleeding has stopped.

Risks

Having a surgical abortion can put you at risk of infection in the fallopian tubes, although many centres will check that you do not already have an infection before you have the operation. You will be asked to return for treatment if you have any signs of infection after the abortion. This is important because infections can reduce your fertility. An abortion can also stretch the cervix so that it becomes 'incompetent'. This is when the opening to the womb is weakened and may not be able to keep in a later and wanted pregnancy. Both these risks are most unlikely with one or two safe and legal abortions which have been done at an early stage of pregnancy.

Can I Have an Abortion?

The health risks of a continued pregnancy and childbirth do outweigh those of a legal abortion carried out under proper medical conditions. However, there is a small risk with any abortion.

No-one ever takes abortion lightly or sees it as an easy option, and you may find the decision whether or not to ask for one to be quite difficult. Abortions are also not always easy to obtain. Your doctor may find it difficult, for moral or medical reasons, to agree to refer you to a hospital or clinic, although if this is so, you should be referred to another doctor. There may not be provision in your area for an NHS service. You may find a private abortion expensive or difficult to obtain.

Where Can I Get Help About Having an Abortion?

If you want an abortion, you will need to see your own family doctor or a doctor at a family planning clinic as soon as possible and ask for advice and help. An abortion can only be done on premises licensed by the Department of Health, such as a hospital or a clinic specially equipped to perform them.

Your own family doctor or a doctor at a youth advisory or at some family planning clinics can send you to a NHS hospital for an abortion. However, NHS abortions may not be available in your area. You may have, or choose, to go to one of the birth control charities who run licensed clinics that provide abortion services. You can go directly to one (see Useful Addresses) or through your doctor or a clinic.

You should be sent quickly for an appointment at a hospital or clinic. If there is any delay you should consider going elsewhere for help. Your own doctor and the surgeon will need to see you for an internal examination and to ask you about your own and your family's health. Both doctors will then have to sign a special form to allow you to have the operation and so will need to justify your reasons for qualifying for an abortion. You do not *need* your partner's permission.

Afterwards

You can get pregnant in the cycle following an abortion, or soon after giving birth. You may like to discuss future contraceptive needs with the doctor, nurse or counsellor with whom you discuss your options before making your final decision.

CHAPTER TEN

Future Contraception

There are several contraceptive methods 'on the drawing board' that may be available in the foreseeable future. There are also some methods that sound interesting but that have in-built problems that appear difficult to overcome.

Reversible Sterilization

Sterilization is the most effective method with the fewest side effects. So a way of using sterilization *and* being able to return to having babies would be a boon. Various methods are being tried. One is to inject a small amount of a plastic that sets to form a plug into the fallopian tubes or the vas. This plug acts as a barrier, stopping sperm and egg from meeting. When a pregnancy is wanted, a small operation can remove the plug. The difficulty is in making the plug effective enough to prevent pregnancy, yet gentle enough to leave no scars that might prevent a return to fertility when it was removed.

Another method is a reversible vasectomy where a section of the vas is removed and replaced with a tiny tube that contains a valve. This valve can be closed to form a barrier to sperm. When a pregnancy is desired, a small operation would reopen the valve and allow sperm to once more travel down the vas. After a pregnancy has been established, another small operation could return the valve to the closed position.

Immunization

If you are immune to an illness, this means that you are

protected from it. Our bodies have an inborn defence against illness, called the immune system, that causes cells and chemicals to break down and throw out anything that could harm us. Immunization is a way of encouraging this system to work against some diseases. If you introduce a very small amount of diphtheria into the body, for instance, the immune system springs into action and builds defences. If you then come into contact fully with diphtheria, the body would have its defences ready to combat it.

With immunization against pregnancy, the body is encouraged to build defences against the hormones normally produced after fertilization. Once immunized against pregnancy, the body rejects any fertilized egg and the egg is then flushed out of the body, as many are quite normally. It is estimated, for instance, that as many as six out of 10 pregnancies never grow to term as the egg fails to implant and is lost as a 'late period'. When a pregnancy *is* planned, the idea is to reverse the immunization. This method is still in the early stages of study.

The Male Pill

A male Pill has been under discussion for years. The main problem is that the hormones that encourage production of sperm are also involved in the man's sex drive. If you try to stop the production of sperm, you can also interfere with the man's sexual desires or ability. You can stop ovulation or egg production in a woman because it is part of the natural process that this only happens at intervals and at times ceases altogether – for instance, during pregnancy, breastfeeding or after the menopause. But sperm production is meant to be a continuous process. Methods which stop sperm being produced may either be dangerous to the man's health or not be reversible. Studies continue.

Hormonal Patches

Skin patches have been used for some time to deliver drugs for heart disease or for hormone replacement therapy. Some drugs will pass slowly into the body if a special patch that is soaked in the liquid drug is stuck to the skin. Patches can be a very useful way of delivering a drug because the preparation is taken in over a length of time in a steady amount. This constant intake means that you can use a smaller dose overall. It also means that the drug goes directly into the bloodstream. This removes the already very small risk of illnesses such as liver disease which may be present with oestrogen taken by mouth.

The drawbacks with skin patches being used as contraception is that you must make sure the patch is on *all the time* for it to keep you safe from pregnancy. Skin patches can be rubbed off by clothes or by bedclothes, and in some women can cause irritation. It may do no harm to go for a few hours without hormone replacement therapy, for example, but the effect could wear off fairly quickly if the patch was a contraceptive one and you may then be at risk of pregnancy. Also, the patch is obvious when you undress and some people might find this embarrassing or inconvenient. Patches may be generally available in the near future.

Female Barrier Methods

There are also various versions of the female condom under discussion. One is like a pair of bikini pants with a soft tube replacing the crotch. This lies folded against the vulva until you have sex, when, with fingers or an erect penis, you push the tube inside to line the vagina. This too may be available in the near future.

CHAPTER ELEVEN

Getting Contraception

Where to Go

For some methods of contraception, you need to see a doctor. All hormonal contraception (the combined and progestogen-only pill, implants, the contraceptive injection and the vaginal ring), the IUD, emergency contraception and male and female sterilization can only be obtained when you have seen and talked to a doctor. Some methods of contraception (such as the diaphragm, cap and natural methods) you *could* obtain or work out how to use on your own, but advice and initial training from someone qualified is vital for effective use. Some methods (male and female condoms, spermicides and sponge) are easily obtained over the counter. But for the most effective use, you may like to see a doctor, nurse or counsellor for information, discussion and teaching that could help you feel confident about using the method.

You can go to your own GP or family doctor for contraception. If you don't want to go to your own doctor for your contraception but want to stay on as his or her patient for other matters, you have the right to visit another doctor just for contraception. Many GPs will offer this service and you could find one near you by asking your local Family Health Services Authority (which oversees family doctors) or Community Health Council (the consumers' watchdog on all health services). Their addresses will be in your local phone book. You would also find lists in main Post Offices and libraries. Or you could go to a family planning clinic near to where you live or work, or to a youth advisory centre such as Brook Advisory Centres – details from your local Health Authority,

Community Health Council, Citizens Advice Bureaux or from the Family Planning Association.

If you need emergency contraception, it is important that you be seen as soon as possible, so ask for an immediate appointment and say why. If your own doctor does not offer this service, or you can't get an appointment quickly enough and your family planning clinic doesn't have a session in time, you can try another GP or the Accident and Emergency department of your local hospital. Genitourinary Medicine Clinics may also be able to help. These are usually listed under Genitourinary Medicine (GUM), Venereal Disease (VD) or Sexually Transmitted Disease (STD) Clinics in your local phone book, often under the main heading of Health Services in your area. You don't need an appointment or a doctor's letter for either a hospital or clinic visit.

Sterilization operations must be done by a doctor qualified in this area in a proper clinic. First you need to see your own family doctor or a doctor at a family planning clinic to be referred for a NHS sterilization. Or you could ask your own doctor to refer you to a private surgeon, or go directly to one of the charities offering birth control services (see Useful Addresses).

Is Contraception Free?

All hormonal methods of contraception, IUDs, diaphragms and caps, spermicides and emergency methods of contraception, are available free from a family doctor, a family planning clinic or a youth advisory centres. In addition, the clinics and centres offer free male and female condoms. The sponge is available free from some family planning clinics. Male and female sterilization may be available free on the National Health Service in your area, but you may find provision is limited only to particular cases, or there could be a waiting list.

Although, therefore, it is not necessary to pay for contraception in the UK, you may choose to do so. Male condoms are on sale in most pharmacies, supermarkets, garages and many local stores or clothing or beauty shops and by mail order. The female condom is available from some shops and supermarkets and mail order, as well as being found with diaphragms and caps, spermicides and the sponge at most pharmacies. Male and female sterilizations may be done privately, either through one of the birth control charities or at a private clinic or hospital. Some family doctors themselves now offer private vasectomies in their own surgeries.

Going to a Doctor for Contraception

If you go to see your doctor about hormonal contraception, the IUD, diaphragms and caps or emergency methods, you will be offered a physical examination. Your weight and your blood pressure will be checked, and you may also be offered a vaginal examination and a cervical smear test. If you are seeing the doctor about hormonal contraception and would prefer to delay having a vaginal examination until a later appointment, this will be fine. However, smear tests are a vital part of health care. They can spot the changes that occur before cancer develops and can allow preventative treatment to be given. Women who have become sexually active should have a smear once every three to five years from the age of 20 to 64. The physical checks made are to be certain that you have no health problems that might affect your use of the method of contraception you have chosen. They are also a routine part of good health care that everybody could benefit from having. A visit to a doctor for contraceptive advice is a very good time to introduce such a routine.

Vaginal Examinations and Smear Tests

For a vaginal examination, you will be asked to remove your lower clothing and to lie down on a couch with knees bent,

your feet flat on the couch and your legs relaxed and open.
Or you may be asked to lie on your side, with your knees bent.
A speculum will then be inserted. This is an instrument made
of plastic or metal. It is designed to gently hold apart the walls
of the vagina, which are usually held collapsed shut and
touching each other. The speculum is made up of two long,
flat, scoop-shaped bowls, hinged at the end in a ring. It looks
rather like a duck's bill. The doctor will often put some
lubricating cream on the end to make insertion easier. With the
bowls held closed, the end of the speculum is inserted into the
vagina and gently eased inside.

The hinge is then operated and the ends moved gently apart,
pushing aside the vaginal walls. This brings the length of your
vagina, the cervix and the end of the vagina into clear view.
Your cervix can then be examined for any signs of abnormal
discharge or for any problems. A smear test will then be taken,
when a few cells are collected from the surface of the cervix.
Cells are collected by gently wiping the shaped end of a
wooden or plastic spatula across the cervix. A small brush may
be inserted gently into the cervical canal to get a full sampling
of cells. These cells are smeared onto a glass slide and the
result is doused in a liquid to 'fix' or preserve it. The slide is
then sent away to a specialized laboratory, usually in a local
hospital, for examination. Results may take six weeks or more
to come back.

After taking a smear, the doctor will remove the speculum
and feel inside your vagina, to make sure everything feels
normal. This internal examination is often called a 'bimanual'
or two-handed examination. With the fingers of one hand the
doctor feels inside your vagina, while the other is placed on
your lower abdomen. By pressing together, the doctor can feel
your internal pelvic organs between the two hands. If you can
imagine feeling around inside a handbag while wearing gloves
and trying to identify your purse or keys or make-up, you can
understand what the doctor is trying to do. The doctor will be
able to tell whether you have any problems by feeling whether
your organs have their characteristic shape, size and texture

and whether they move as freely as they should. The doctor will probably ask if you have any pain and will watch your face as he or she does this internal examination to tell, from your expression, whether you feel any pain or discomfort.

As well as doing an internal examination, the doctor is likely to take the opportunity to examine your breasts. You will be asked to remove the top half of your clothes and the doctor will look at both breasts and nipples. The doctor will then press the flats of his or her fingers all over your breasts and into the armpit, to make sure your breasts feel normal. This examination is often done twice – once standing and once lying down, as some lumps will only become apparent in one but not the other position.

You will also need to discuss your own health and the health of your relatives. This is because certain conditions, in you or your family, are 'absolute contraindications' to – that is, if you have that condition it is important you must not be given – some methods of contraception. Others may not prevent you from having a particular method of contraception but may mean you and your doctor should take particular care. It is important you and your doctor discuss any problems that are relevant.

Useful Addresses

Family Planning Association
27-35 Mortimer Street
London W1N 7RJ
Tel: 071 636 7866

The FPA in Wales
Grace Phillips House
4 Museum Place
Cardiff CF1 3BG
Tel: 0222 342766

The FPA in Northern Ireland
113 University Street
Belfast BT7 1HP
Tel: 0232 325488

**International Planned
Parenthood Federation**
Regent's College
Inner Circle
Regent's Park
London NW1 4NS
Tel: 071 486 0741

**Brook Advisory Centres
(Head Office)**
153a East Street
London SE17 2SD
Tel: 071 708 1234

Health Education Authority
Hamilton House
Mabledon Place
London WC1H 9TX
Tel: 071 383 3833

**BPAS (British Pregnancy
Advisory Service)**
Austy Manor
Wootton Wawen
Solihull
West Midlands B95 6DA
Tel: 0564 793225

Pregnancy Advisory Service
13 Charlotte Street
London W1P 1HD
Tel: 071 637 8962

Marie Stopes House
108 Whitfield Street
London W1P 6BE
Tel: 071 388 0662

LIFE
LIFE House
1a Newbold Terrace
Leamington Spa
Warwicks CV32 4EA
Tel: 0926 421587

British Agencies for Adoption and Fostering
11 Southwark Street
London SE1 1RG
Tel: 071 409 8800

National Childbirth Trust
Alexander House
Oldham Terrace
London W3 6NH
Tel: 081 992 8637

National Council for One Parent Families
255 Kentish Town Road
London NW5 2LX
Tel: 071 267 1361

British Association for Counselling
1 Regent Place
Rugby
Warwicks CV21 2PJ
Tel: 0788 578328/9

Relate
Herbert Gray College
Little Church Street
Rugby CV21 3AP
Tel: 0788 73241

The Natural Family Planning Service
Catholic Marriage Advisory Council
Clitherow House
1 Blythe Mews
Blythe Road
London W14 0NW
Tel: 071 371 1341

The Natural Family Planning Unit
Birmingham Maternity Hospital
Queen Elizabeth Medical Centre
Birmingham B15 2TG
Tel: 021 472 1377

Women's Health Concern
PO Box 1629
London W8 6AU
Tel: 071 938 3932

Women's Health
52 Featherstone Street
London EC1Y 8RT
Tel: 071 251 6580

Index